Conquer Your Diabetes: Prevention • Control • Remission

Advance Praise

Two expert authors have written a clearly articulated patient-focused tour de force on the complex disorder of diabetes. Afflicting almost half a billion people worldwide, this silent metabolic disorder has crept into all our lives as a silent adversary to multiple body systems. Importantly, this book amplifies how the health impact of diabetes extends far beyond control of blood sugar levels. The broad spectrum and magnitude of adverse targeting of kidney, heart, vascular, retina, bone, reproductive, immune, gastrointestinal, neurologic, and psychologic dysfunctions are emphasized as determinants of disease, healthcare utilization, cost and economic and societal burdens.

Ranging from beautifully crafted and colorful historic perspectives, all the way through disease epidemiology, symptoms, signs, multiple management approaches, newest medications, cutting edge technologies for insulin delivery systems, and transplantation, each chapter remains keenly focused on patient and family well-being while coping with this lifelong metabolic dysfunction. Importantly, special life situations like surgery, pregnancy and exercise are covered with both patient sensitivity and scientific accuracy. This is a wonderful and essential volume of enduring value to be enjoyed and referred to by patients, loved ones, nurses, educators, physicians, public health experts, as well as trainees and all those engaged in scholarly discovery for this all-encompassing metabolic disorder of our times.

—Shlomo Melmed, MB, ChB
Dean and Executive Vice President,
Professor of Medicine,
Cedars Sinai Medical Center
Los Angeles, CA

Preventing diabetes and its complications must be one of the highest priorities of any country. Singapore declared war against diabetes in 2016, mobilizing the whole of society to address one of the biggest challenges to our resources. In this effort, nothing is more important than clear, accurate, and understandable information. Professors Abrahamson and Chopra have given the world a priceless guide. Whatever your background, I am confident that you will find this book invaluable. This needs to be translated into as many languages as possible for all to benefit.

—John E. L. Wong, MBBS, FAMS, FRCP, FACP
Isabel Chan Professor in Medical Sciences
Senior Vice President (Health Innovation and Translation)
The National University of Singapore, and
Senior Advisor, The National University Health System, Singapore

There are few other diseases where the patient's role is so critical to living in good health and avoiding complications. This wonderful guide to self-care from two very experienced clinicians will be an important tool for those wanting to do their best. The book is full of practical and sage advice as well as useful tips and tricks that are hard to find elsewhere.

—Abraham Verghese, MD
Professor of Medicine, Stanford University, and
Author of "Cutting for Stone"

Climbing Everest and walking to the Poles as a patient with diabetes was a tremendous challenge. Significant developments in healthcare and medicine made the journeys possible. This new book examines these milestones and, equally importantly, the emotional toll of an impending condition.

Predictable and stable insulin at temperature has been a huge help. Convenient, rapid and accurate blood testing has also contributed to my success. Hemoglobin A1c results add to the ever-changing circumstances of adventure by indicating stable insulin, diet and exercise over time. A better understanding of diet and glycogen was of particular aid when preparing for the South Pole and developing the life-sustaining rations. Emotional vulnerability has also been examined by the authors and plays a daily role in diabetes management and for those that we love. After 45 years as a "type 1," my very existence rests on these medical breakthroughs. I highly recommend this read.

—Will Cross
7 Summits & 2 Poles

This book, written by two renowned Professors at Harvard Medical School is one which every patient with diabetes, needs to read. I personally have seen the destruction the disease has had on the Latino Community. It's a malady afflicting millions worldwide. This book will inform and inspire the reader that there is hope. Dr. Sanjiv Chopra and Dr. Martin Abrahamson have written with exceptional clarity and compassion a fantastic book. This book is filled with advice to help you or your loved ones to lead happy, healthy, and more fulfilled lives.

—Edward James Olmos
Actor, Director, Producer and Activist

It is very likely you have heard the words 'This book is a "Must Read."' Well, this excellent book 'Conquer Your Diabetes' by two renowned Harvard Medical School Professors, Drs. Martin Abrahamson and Sanjiv Chopra, is definitely a "Must Read."

What I liked particularly about this book was that the authors adopted an evidence-based approach delivering what they believe that you, as the reader, would like to know and what they thought you should know! The advice and information they have offered should guide you through your day-to-day activities to manage your diabetes.

Their book provides a well-balanced contribution of up-to-date information on nutrition, exercise, new therapies, surgery for obesity and diabetes, insights regarding the gut microbiome, and technology. And, as well, information on what nearly everyone with diabetes wants to know. This includes what is around the corner including pancreas transplantation, and the latest technological advances in self-blood glucose monitoring and insulin pumps. Yes, it is all there! Even the topic of vaccinations assumes importance in the context of the COVID-19 pandemic with nations around the world and scientists in the race for this critical viral attack.

Many decades ago, Dr. Wilfrid G. Oakley, a famous English diabetes physician, said: "Man may be the captain of his fate, but he is also the victim of his blood sugar". These were the "not so good old days" for people with diabetes.

But as Bob Dylan's famous song "The Times They Are a-Changin'" goes, by following the excellent advice in this book, you will hold in your hands the "weapon" that can change your destiny by mastering your diabetes.

—Professor Paul Zimmet, AO, MD, PhD, FRACP, FRCP, FTSE
Professor of Diabetes, Monash University
Victorian Senior Australian of the Year 2018

The diagnosis of diabetes is for most, a daunting prospect. People with type 1 diabetes have to learn a vast amount of complex information and then put it into practice every day for the rest of their lives while those with type 2 diabetes are faced with the challenging task of fundamentally changing and maintaining their lifestyle.

In 'Conquer Your Diabetes,' Martin Abrahamson and Sanjiv Chopra demystify diabetes with considerable skill, providing important information in a readable and fascinating way, while at the same time, giving those with the condition the confidence to manage it successfully.

I have no hesitation in recommending it to anyone with diabetes. They will learn a huge amount and enjoy the experience. I congratulate the authors in both recognizing the need for such a book and achieving their aims so effectively.

—Simon Heller, BA, MB, BChir, DM, FRCP
Professor of Clinical Diabetes, University of Sheffield, and
Honorary Consultant Physician, Sheffield Teaching Hospitals, UK

This is an interesting and fun-to-read book that takes stories about patients to create insight into important messages about the pathogenesis and treatment of diabetes and its many complications. Drs. Abrahamson and

Chopra have instilled human qualities to the diabetes teaching, which makes the book appropriate for both patients and physicians.

—C. Ronald Kahn, MD
Past-President and Chief Academic Officer, Joslin Diabetes Center, and Mary K. Iacocca Professor of Medicine, Harvard Medical School

This is a much-needed comprehensive book on everything diabetes. The authors have done an excellent job in producing a book that is easy to read and includes everything anyone needs to know about diabetes from prevention to treatment. I will recommend it to all my patients.

—Anne Peters, MD
Director, USC Clinical Diabetes Program
Professor of Clinical Medicine, Keck School of Medicine of USC
Author of "Conquer Diabetes" and "The Type 1 Diabetes Self-Care Manual: A Complete Guide to Type 1 Diabetes Across the Lifespan for People with Diabetes, Parents, and Caregivers."

Great practical knowledge and highlights of the many paths that diabetes can throw at its victims, accompanied by treatments for a healthy approach and inspirational anecdotes of success. Due to the new technologies described herein, it is proof positive that you can do anything with diabetes if you set your mind to it. So happy to be back in the air in the driver's seat! Thanks go to Dr. Abrahamson for sticking with me through all these years and the considerable obstacles that have now been removed. From day one of diabetes until now, he has said we can get you back to flying - Success!

—Captain Mike Jackson
B767 Airline Pilot

Control and mastery of diabetes is now in your hands! This easy-to-understand book will empower you with tools and activities to give you a healthier and more fulfilling life AND includes the future of caring for (and maybe curing) your diabetes!

—Frank J. Domino, MD
Professor and Family Physician, University of Massachusetts Medical School

If you are a person with diabetes, this succinct primer by two world-renowned doctors with decades of clinical and research experience gives you the latest information on the disease, how it affects you, what problems may arise, how it can be monitored and kept under control with diet, weight loss, foods, supplements, medications, and lifestyle changes. If you have the early chemical changes of diabetes (pre-diabetes) you can learn strategies to lower the risk of disease progression and even return back to normal.

—Peng Fan, MD
Professor of Medicine, David Geffen School of Medicine, UCLA

This book, written by two eminent physicians with nearly 100 years of clinical experience between them, will strike a powerful chord for the reader. It brings the experience of one of the world's most important problems, diabetes, and its impact on our health and lives to the forefront in an understandable and engaging manner. The book takes you on a journey from the history of the disease to the science, to its effect on people's personal stories. Anyone who is a patient and who treats patients will find this book both knowledgeable and useful.

—Panagiota Caralis, MD, JD
Professor of Medicine, Miller School of Medicine, University of Miami, and Medical Director of the Women Veterans Program, Miami Veteran's Health Service

Living with diabetes can be overwhelming. So much to learn, so much to know, so much to change... Knowledge alone will not propel anyone to lead a healthy active life with diabetes. You have to put this knowledge to work to be successful. The tools to be successful are embedded in the learnings in this practical, up-to-date, and readable guide from two respected clinician-teachers. Within these pages, Drs. Abrahamson and Chopra explore all elements of diabetes from clinical presentation to complications; from today's treatments to what might be coming tomorrow. This book will help you better understand diabetes and facilitate your ability to control diabetes rather than letting it control you.

—Alan C. Moses, MD, FACP
Former Professor of Medicine, Harvard Medical School, and
Former Chief Medical Officer of the Joslin Diabetes Center, and
Former Global Chief Medical Officer of Novo Nordisk A/S

Diagnosed with diabetes? Use this book to regain control of your health! Benefit from the extensive expertise of these brilliant Harvard physicians and learn not only about the latest research, but also practical tips, tricks, and tools you need to positively impact and ultimately change the course of your disease. 'Conquer Your Diabetes' will help you understand aspects of your disease far beyond blood sugar, and empower you to have more informed, productive encounters with all your health providers.

—Jill Grimes, MD, FAAFP
Clinical Instructor, University
Massachusetts Medical School
Author of "The ULTIMATE College Student Health Handbook: Your Guide for Everything from Hangovers to Homesickness"

Diabetes is a global pandemic and often a silent killer. Yet, there are so many without the knowledge to master this manageable condition. The renowned authors gift us with more than an easy-to-read book. It provides much needed, science-based practical knowledge for the lay person. If you have diabetes or care for a person with it, this is an essential companion...you can't afford to live without it!

—Venkat Srinivasan, PhD
Co-Founder, KnowYourMeds.com, and
Managing Director, Innospark Ventures

In this accessible compendium of knowledge, two of Harvard's leading physicians-scientists bring to bear their formidable clinical experience, compassion and wisdom to help you navigate the complexity of diabetes. If you choose one resource, make it this gem of a book that is chock-full of information that will inspire and lead you to well-being. 'Conquer Your Diabetes' is further enriched by the stories of people just like you who share practical advice gleamed through the prism of their own successful journeys.

This engaging guide will set you on a path to good health and enable you to become master of your fate.

—Gina Vild
Former Associate Dean at Harvard
Medical School, and
Co-author of "The Two Most Important Days, How to Find your Purpose and Live a Happier, Healthier Life"

Written keeping in mind the needs of the person with diabetes, this book relies on the vast experience and knowledge of two world renown physicians. They have accomplished a phenomenal task: translating science to an intriguing reading. The person with diabetes can find here, page after page, a very up-to-date and yet easy to follow and to understand little encyclopedia covering all aspects of diabetes, including cutting edge research. The information provided is so crispy and immediate that I would suggest this book not to remain within the diabetes community but become an informative reading to the general public and definitely to all who care about health.

—Stefano Del Prato
Professor of Endocrinology, University of
Pisa, Italy

Kudos to the authors who have done great work in offering this timely book. It is current, comprehensive, accessible and should be directly useful to anyone with diabetes!

—Jeffrey S. Flier, MD
Higginson Professor of Medicine &
former Dean, Harvard Medical School

Drs. Abrahamson and Chopra have done a masterful job in creating an invaluable resource that should be read by all patients with diabetes, their families, and anyone interested in learning about this disease that affects more than 460 million people worldwide. What is remarkable are the ways that they have seamlessly integrated scholarship with readability, presented both evidence-based information and illustrative patient cases, and blended an historical perspective with the most up to date, cutting edge knowledge about all aspects of the disease and its treatment. Their approach has been comprehensive, and the material presented in a fashion that well demonstrates why both authors are most highly regarded as world-class clinicians and educators.

—Steven Weinberger, MD, MACP, FRCP
Executive Vice President and CEO
Emeritus, American College of
Physicians, and
Adjunct Professor of Medicine, Perelman
School of Medicine at the University of
Pennsylvania

As I read through this comprehensive book on diabetes, I was impressed with the breadth and depth of the content. Drs. Abrahamson and Chopra have managed to integrate history, real cases, extensive new research, and very practical pointers throughout the entire book. So inspiring and lovely! Tackling issues such as gut microbiomes, insulin formulations and so many dietary approaches, they have made sense of all of these complex issues and provide relevant pointers and pull-outs for the reader. My most sincere congratulations to Drs. Abrahamson and Chopra for a truly unique contribution to our world of diabetes.

—Athena Philis-Tsimikas, MD
Corporate Vice President, Scripps
Whittier Diabetes Institute

'Conquer Your Diabetes' is a superb compendium for both patients and the general public. It provides a critical review of the clinical presentations of diabetes as well as generalizable review of the causes of this significant disease. Additionally, preventive strategies, current therapies and the future of diabetes treatments are explored in significant details. Most importantly, Drs. Abrahamson and Chopra have created a platform to make all aspects of diabetes accessible to everyone.

—Anthony N. Hollenberg, MD
Sanford I. Weill Chair
Joan and Sanford I. Weill Department of Medicine, and
Professor of Medicine, Weill Cornell Medicine, and
Physician-in-Chief, New York-Presbyterian Hospital/Weill Cornell Medical Center

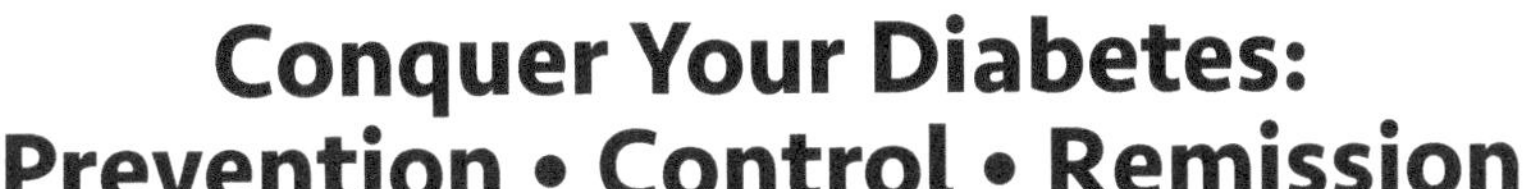

Conquer Your Diabetes: Prevention • Control • Remission

Dr. Martin Abrahamson & Dr. Sanjiv Chopra

With a foreword by Deepak Chopra, MD

Abrahamson Chopra Publishing

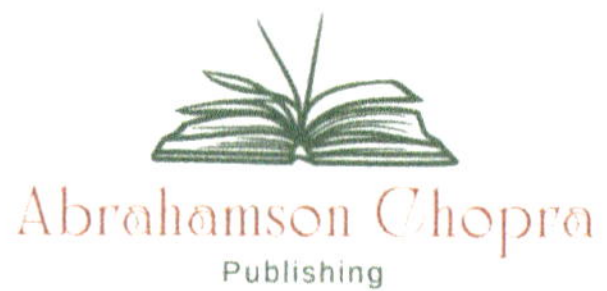

Abrahamson Chopra Publishing

www.conqueryourdiabetes.com

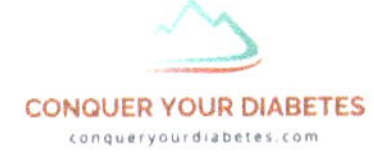

The information provided in this book is current at the time of publication. However, medical knowledge and practice advance at a rapid rate. This book aims to provide accurate, authoritative information about diabetes. However, the information provided here is for educational purposes only and does not substitute for professional medical advice. We suggest you check with your primary care clinician and consultants involved in your care before making any changes in your diet, exercise regimen or medications.

Neither the publisher nor the authors assume any liability for any injury and/or damage to persons or property arising from or related to use of material in this book.

ISBN: 979-8-9854237-1-6

Dedications

I dedicate this book to Sunita Vadehra, my sister-in-law, for inspiring me and so many others with her brilliance, compassion, wit, creativity, love, courage and resilience. And I honor Amol Vadehra (1977–2015), a brilliant, creative and luminous soul who brought pure laughter and so much joy into the lives of countless people. And to Mallika Vadehra, a beautiful and compassionate person.

SC

I dedicate this book to my wife Sharon, a devoted wife, mother, grandmother and daughter; and to my children, Talia, Adam, Darren, Daniela, Nicky, and Dan; and to my nine grandchildren who bring unbridled joy and luminous light into my and so many other lives. And to my late parents, Abe and Anita Abrahamson, whose never-ending love, support, and encouragement has meant the world to me.

MA

The diabetic who knows the most, lives the longest.

—Elliot P. Joslin, MD

Preface

It is not the mountain we conquer, but ourselves.

—Sir Edmund Hillary, the first person to climb Mount Everest with Tenzing Norgay in 1953

We wrote this book to inform and empower people with diabetes, those at risk for diabetes, and all their loved ones affected, to help them live full and fulfilling lives.

When someone has a chronic medical disorder, the illness should not define them. And with all the scientific advances in the management of diabetes, an individual can scale any heights.

William H. Cross is a mountain climber who developed type 1 diabetes in 1976 at the age of 9. In May 2006, he reached the top of Mount Everest. In addition, he has climbed the highest mountains on all seven continents and trekked to both the North and South Poles. His story is inspiring, and a tribute to his incredible tenacity, but also to the medical treatment he has received. In the fifteen years since, there have been phenomenal advances in our understanding of diabetes, with its myriad nuances, technological breakthroughs in monitoring blood glucose levels, and in novel treatments, both medical and surgical.

In this book we inform the reader of how they can leverage these advances to control their diabetes and, in some cases, to even cause the diabetes to go into remission. We also recommend strategies that can help individuals with prediabetes from developing full-fledged diabetes. We share stories of many of our patients, who have done this and inspired us and countless numbers of our colleagues.

Diabetes is a major health issue whose global prevalence has reached alarming levels. It is a major cause of morbidity and mortality. In 2000, there were an estimated 150 million adults with diabetes in the world. In 2019, there were an estimated 465 million. By 2030, this number will grow to almost 580 million, and in 2045, to 700 million. Almost 95% of these people have type 2 diabetes, the remainder have type 1 diabetes.

Worldwide, an astounding 50% of people with type 2 diabetes have not been diagnosed.

Currently it is estimated that there are almost 375 million people with prediabetes in the world. This means that millions more are at risk for the development of diabetes if appropriate measures are not undertaken. In aggregate, in 2020, more than three quarters of a billion people in the world either have or are at risk for the development of diabetes. About 1.1 million children and adolescents aged under 20 years have type 1 diabetes. Alarmingly, an increasing number of children and adolescents are being diagnosed with type 2 diabetes, primarily because of the increase in the prevalence of obesity throughout the world.

Diabetes is a disorder that can affect virtually every organ of the body. It is a serious threat to global health with no respect for socioeconomic status, ethnicity, gender, or national boundaries. The potential for life-threatening complications leads to an increased cost in managing this one medical disorder. If not controlled, people with diabetes experience a much greater need for medical care, a higher risk of hospitalization and premature death, and a reduction in quality of life and undue stress on themselves and their loved ones. Globally, diabetes is amongst the top 10 causes of mortality, with 4 million deaths attributable to diabetes in 2019.

The costs related to diabetes are astronomical. A few years ago, health expenditure on diabetes was estimated to be $760 billion. This is estimated to reach $825 billion by 2030 and does not include other costs resulting from loss of productivity, absenteeism from work, premature disability, and mortality.

In this book, we offer you tools and strategies to tackle this chronic condition and live a longer and healthier life. Remember that diabetes does not define who you are and what you can do. Rather, you can master your diabetes and be a beacon of hope and inspiration to others.

To quote the English poet William Ernest Henley (1849–1903):

"I am the master of my fate: I am the captain of my soul."

Martin Abrahamson & Sanjiv Chopra

January 2022

Foreword by Deepak Chopra, MD

A revolution in wellness is occurring all around us, and it is high time that the revolution reached diabetes. The first half of that sentence is indisputable. The movement toward self-care is probably the single biggest shift in modern medicine. It has occurred outside the medical schools, doctors' offices, research labs and massive drug companies. The movement is fueled by a single inspiring ideal: lifelong well-being.

I'll comment further on this ideal and why we should all adopt it. But first to the second part of the opening sentence. It is high time that the wellness revolution reached diabetes. This will be news to millions of people who leave diabetes out of their lifestyle choices. They pay daily attention to what they eat. They are conscious of gaining weight or being under too much stress. They probably have some idea of the risk of heart disease and stroke connected to cholesterol.

By comparison, diabetes gets almost no attention until someone has arrived at the stage where symptoms appear, and it is time to see the doctor. That's not good enough, and to provide a shift into wellness and self-care, the authors of this book have acted with urgency, compassion, and immense experience to provide the one book everyone should read who has the slightest interest in lifelong well-being.

The fact is that diabetes has arrived at our doorstep, and it has come almost silently. As Drs. Martin Abrahamson and Sanjiv Chopra, two world-renowned professors at Harvard Medical School, point out, more than 460 million people in the world already have diabetes. By 2045 that number will reach 700 million, and almost the same number of people will have prediabetes, a condition that predisposes someone to acquiring diabetes over the next ten years. These sobering figures are likely to keep rising, in large part due to our sedentary lifestyle and poor nutrition. The correlation between type 2 diabetes and obesity is also seriously troubling.

Once a threat is pointed out and risks are assessed, the road to overcoming the threat should be open. But it isn't. One thing medicine has learned in the age of prevention, which is nearly five decades old, is that fear is a poor motivator. No one can live comfortably with a constant danger, and so we turn to those false friends, denial and distraction. We ignore the trouble facing us, and we run to find something that will take our minds off our worries.

This is where Abrahamson and Chopra bring new light to the whole field of self-care and diabetes. Their book is about lifelong wellness, even in the face of being diagnosed with the disease. The most inspiring chapter here is titled "Patients as Teachers," which recounts the stories of remarkable people who have lived for decades with diabetes, leading healthy, fulfilling lives. No matter which side of the stethoscope you find yourself on, diabetes respects no boundaries. It strikes in every society, ethnic group, and income level. That isn't news, but many would be surprised by something Dr. Abrahamson says at the outset of "Patients as Teachers":

> *I have seen the illiterate rural laborer with type 1 diabetes who has no access to electricity take superb care of himself and maintain excellent glucose control; and I have also seen a highly intelligent and wealthy entrepreneur unable to adhere to a treatment regimen of primarily diet and exercise and develop multiple complications.*

From such experiences, the authors have arrived at a wise conclusion: Every patient must be given individualized treatment. We all respond to a diagnosis, or potential threats to our well-being, according to complex factors that make us unique. Self-care must therefore be based on self-awareness. You will gain an abundance of information in this rewarding book. But more importantly, you can use it as a mirror in which to see yourself.

Lifelong well-being is such a new prospect, even in the most advanced societies, that everyone is feeling their way with a mixture of hoping, wishing, deciding, resisting, and complying. The crucial thing is to have a vision of the goal. The vision as applied to diabetes is provided here in every detail. It is up to each of us to adopt the vision and make it our own. That's a universal message when it comes to wellness. If you want your wellness to include mastery over diabetes, this book is a must-read.

Deepak Chopra

Acknowledgements

We gratefully acknowledge Amanda Annis for shepherding us during the initial writing of this book. Her wise counsel and suggestions undoubtedly made this book more robust and readable.

We acknowledge with gratitude Dr. Alan Moses, a dear friend and colleague, who read the initial manuscript word by word and provided us with invaluable suggestions that we duly incorporated.

We are indebted to Paul Mayhew for his innumerable suggestions on how to make this book easier to read by incorporating simple illustrations and tables, and for his diligent and dedicated role as project manager for this book.

A sincere thank you to all our colleagues and friends who took the time read the advanced copy of the book and endorse it so favorably and eloquently.

And last, but by no means least, we are humbled and grateful for what our patients have taught us. Their stories, many of which are included in this book, continue to inspire us.

Contents

I

HOW PATIENTS MASTER THEIR DIABETES

Attitude is a little thing that makes a big difference.

—Winston Churchill

Winners never quit, and quitters never win.

—Vince Lombardi

I, Martin Abrahamson, have had the privilege of helping people manage their diabetes for many years, initially in South Africa where I trained and then practiced for some years, and subsequently in Boston, USA. I have developed long-lasting relationships with many of my patients, getting to know them, their spouses or significant others and their children and grandchildren, to become a friend with "special knowledge," rather than solely their "doctor."

Diabetes is a condition that has no social, economic, or political boundaries. It affects people from all ethnic groups, although there is a higher prevalence in Asian Americans, Pacific Islanders, Native Americans and Hispanic people compared to others. It affects the rich, the poor, people with doctorates, and the illiterate. It affects successful entrepreneurs, academics, blue-collar workers, manual laborers, people who live in rural areas, and people who live in cities. Each person with diabetes has his or her unique challenges with which they must live every day.

Universal Disease, Individual Treatment

Clinicians who take care of people with diabetes need to understand everyone's unique circumstances, and that he or she is living with a chronic condition 24 hours a day, 7 days a week, 365 days a year. This applies to people with both type 1 diabetes and type 2 diabetes.

Because of each patient's unique circumstances, I, like many of my peers have recognized that treatment needs to be individualized, something which we have articulated throughout this book. At the same time, I have also realized that, despite all the efforts made to help some people manage their diabetes, the responses to recommendations, motivation to improve or maintain good glucose control and the degree of "engagement" varies enormously from person to person and is not related to social or economic circumstances. It also varies at different times of years (holidays being a common example) and with changes in life circumstances (loss of job, illness of family members, etc.).

I have seen the illiterate rural laborer with type 1 diabetes who has no access to electricity take superb care of himself and maintain excellent glucose control; and I have also seen a highly intelligent and wealthy entrepreneur, unable to adhere to a treatment regimen of primarily diet and exercise interventions, unfortunately go on to develop multiple serious complications.

The challenges that people face are demanding. Some patients' stories are truly remarkable! I have learned an enormous amount from people with diabetes whom I have cared for and have been able to use this invaluable knowledge to help many others. Many of my patients are incredible teachers and amazing sources of inspiration. We have aimed to imbue in this book as much of this knowledge and inspiration as we could. But, below, I am going to share two stories that we hope will particularly encourage you to meet the challenges that you face day-to-day, month-to-month and year-to-year.

KH: Living Life to the Fullest

I first met KH when she was 73 years of age. She had already had type 1 diabetes for 65 years having been diagnosed at the age of eight in 1937. I was privileged to take care of her in the latter part of her life, until she passed away six months after her 90th birthday, having lived with type 1 diabetes for 82 years.

At the time of her diagnosis, she was living in a small town called Paris, 60 miles from Toronto, Ontario. She was hospitalized for ten days at the Sick Children's Hospital in Toronto and started on insulin – this was only 15 years after insulin had become available. At that time there was only 1 kind of insulin – regular porcine insulin. It had to be injected with reusable syringes and needles. The needles were much larger and longer than the ones we use today and certainly caused more discomfort. Additionally, the needles and syringes had to be boiled to sterilize them after each use, and the insulin needles needed to be sharpened regularly using a sharpening stone! As the insulin then was less concentrated, the volume injected was much higher than modern preparations. Not only this, but it also contained many impurities which caused local skin reactions.

KH was homeschooled after being diagnosed. She described her mother as being "highly protective." Her mother weighed all her food and carefully monitored her intake. She injected her insulin four times a day and tested her urine for glucose multiple times a day. This was done by adding a special solution called Benedict's solution to the urine and then boiling the mixture on a gas flame in the kitchen. The color change that ensued reflected the amount of glucose in the urine. Home blood glucose monitoring did not exist at that time (it became available in the 1970s), nor were there HbA1c measurements (which also became available in the 1970s).

KH often reminded me how her mother would massage her hips with cocoa butter prior to injecting the insulin. Initially, her life was socially isolated, and she was not able to go to sleepovers or birthday parties. She was not allowed any sweets and she said, "my life was that of a protected, pampered invalid." She described how this lack of freedom affected her feelings of self-worth and how she had to fight to regain confidence in later years. However, she also commented that her mother had taught her self-discipline that would stand her in good stead for the rest of her life.

When she started college, she was not allowed to leave home. She commuted by bus every day to Waterloo College, 30 miles from home. Ultimately, she transferred to the University of Western Ontario and lived in the dorms there.

She recounted how doctors would tell her that she could expect to live a much shorter life span than many others, and that some doctors advised her to marry a man with children because the "chances of having your own (baby) are nil." She married in 1953. She had a devoted husband who was incredibly supportive and who helped her resolve her feelings of "isolation." She described her first pregnancy and how she was told how risky it would be and how unlikely it was that she would deliver a live infant. The baby was born prematurely at Toronto General Hospital and required intensive nursing but thankfully survived. She subsequently had two more children after leaving Canada and relocating to the United States.

Diabetes did not stop her from enjoying an active life – she took up aerobics, and exercised frequently, and in later years she took up curling and represented the United States in an international curling event. She lived to see many advances in diabetes management and embraced them all – she started using disposable syringes and testing blood glucoses at home in the 1970s, started using human insulin and then insulin analogues in the 1980s and 1990s. She embraced the use of insulin pen devices when these became available and started using continuous glucose monitoring when this became available a few years before she passed away.

She suffered numerous setbacks and complications, but this did not deter her from leading an active life and traveling with her husband throughout the USA and to all corners of the world. She broke multiple bones and required treatment for osteoporosis. She developed celiac disease, a disease with a higher incidence in those with type 1 diabetes, in her late 40s, and had to maintain a gluten-free diet. She described vividly how her symptoms of celiac disease flummoxed doctors for many months. "I had chronic diarrhea, gas and allergic lesions under my arms," she told us, and then added, "My weight was dropping, I had broken capillaries on my legs, inflamed gums and aching teeth." She also described frequent episodes of nocturnal diarrhea that doctors thought was a complication of her diabetes. Finally, she said, her diabetologist at the time referred her to a gastroenterologist who did a biopsy that confirmed the diagnosis of celiac disease. "My villi were flat against the lining of my intestines!" she commented.

Her diabetes led to retinopathy (retinal disease of the eye) that required laser photocoagulation. She was treated for osteoporosis and had numerous falls leading to several broken bones over the years, including her clavicle and leg. She developed coronary artery disease and had several heart attacks, but she remained active physically and mentally and lived life to the fullest.

When her husband died in 2010, she was devastated. She had been married for 58 years and had felt totally dependent on him. But, she said, "I rallied." She recalled the discipline her mother had instilled in her during her formative years, and was determined to manage on her own, which she did for the next ten years.

She never "gave up" and was truly an inspiration. I was privileged to participate in her care for nearly 20 years. In 2015, she delivered an address at the annual American Diabetes Association meeting and concluded by saying, "I have had a pretty full life despite the diabetes. I am still curling and exercising, and I keep my mind sharp by analyzing stocks!"

At an annual Update in Internal Medicine course that I co-direct with Dr. Chopra, she told this story to more than 500 physicians from all over the USA and more than 45 countries. She received a standing ovation – a fitting tribute to her tenacity and courage!

The challenges that face people with type 2 diabetes who are overweight or obese are not necessarily the same as those that people with type 1 diabetes must face. For people who have type 2 diabetes and are overweight or obese, lifestyle modification is a major challenge. It is not easy to lose weight and maintain weight loss indefinitely. It requires a lot of motivation and determination.

LS: Learning to Prioritize Health

LS is a patient of mine who was referred by his primary care physician because he had developed the classic symptoms of diabetes: his blood glucose was almost 500 mg/dL and his hemoglobin A1c (HbA1c) was 16.9%!

> **Hemoglobin A1c (HbA1c)** is a blood test that reflects one's average blood glucose over the preceding 90 days (see page 140).

He told me that his doctor had, for many years, "been at me to lose weight." But he went on, "I am a busy professional, and can't find time to exercise, or pay any attention to what I eat." When I met LS, he had gained over 60 pounds [27 kg] over the previous ten years but had already lost nearly 20 pounds [9 kg]. I told him he needed to start insulin because his glucose levels were so high, and he told me that he would do whatever he could to come off insulin, that he was going to "turn my life around." We agreed that this was possible, provided he committed to change his lifestyle, i.e., lose weight by watching his caloric intake, eating healthier foods, and starting to exercise regularly. He started insulin and metformin treatment.

Three months later he had lost almost 40 pounds [18 kg], his HbA1c had dropped to 6.1%, and we could stop his insulin! Impressively, he has maintained this level of glucose control for the past seven years, and, while he has gained a few pounds back, he has remained off insulin, and requires only metformin and a glucagon-like peptide-1 (GLP-1) receptor agonist to help him maintain excellent glucose control. He exercises regularly, watches his carbohydrates carefully, and still manages to lead an active professional life. He has learned how to incorporate – and **maintain** – important components of lifestyle modification into his daily routine.

> LS realized that he needed to make some major lifestyle changes for his own benefit, succeeded in doing so and maintained these efforts. It is never too late to make these changes if one needs to! The long-term benefits are clear!

A Winning Attitude

These are just 2 examples of people who have "risen to the occasion" and taken control of their situation. They have demonstrated tremendous resilience; they have overcome multiple challenges and maintained an upbeat attitude.

In all the years that I saw KH, she did not complain once about her situation, or the challenges she had to face. I calculated that in her 82 years of having diabetes she likely took about 120,000 injections of insulin and pricked her finger almost as many times! She lived a normal life, raised 3 children and traveled the world. She was all about living a successful life with diabetes and not letting diabetes dictate how she lived. This takes work but it is possible. Indeed, with new technologies including insulin pumps and continuous glucose monitoring, people with type 1 diabetes are less and less limited in what they feel that they can do.

We have so many more tools at our disposal today to help us achieve treatment goals. The advances in medical therapies, monitoring tools, and access to healthy foods and scientific proof of the value of exercise and healthy eating have made it easier to do this, and reduce morbidity and mortality from diabetes. But there is one thing that is as important as all of this, and that is an upbeat and courageous attitude where one never gives up.

There are many, many people who take optimal care of their health and lead productive and fulfilling lives. The talented and Oscar-winning actress Halle Berry is one such person. She was diagnosed with diabetes at the age of 22 and was started on insulin as it was thought she had type 1 diabetes. However, she modified her diet, exercises regularly, and is reportedly not taking insulin, which leads us to speculate that she has type 2 diabetes.

Billie Jean King, a famous tennis champion, developed type 2 diabetes when she was 63. She said, "anyone can develop diabetes, even an athlete." King has a family history of diabetes and also had an eating disorder in the past. "I was a binge eater. I don't binge eat anymore, but for about ten years, I was being very cruel to my poor little pancreas."

To keep her condition under control, she exercises frequently, takes her medication regularly, and tests her blood sugar daily.

Randy Jackson, a music producer and former *American Idol* judge, was diagnosed with type 2 diabetes in 2002. At the time he weighed more than 300 pounds [136 kg]. Even though his father had diabetes, Jackson says, he never imagined it would happen to him. Following gastric bypass surgery, he lost approximately 100 pounds. With healthy eating and daily exercise, he has kept his weight off and his diabetes is under control.

These stories continue to inspire us.

Throughout our careers we have often shared such stories, and their valuable lessons, with patients to motivate them to live life to the fullest. We also continue to recount them to clinicians throughout the United States and abroad as we teach, learn and travel. Without fail, we have found that the stories resonate deeply, and our listeners express profound gratitude to us for sharing them. With many of these stories collected in this book, we hope you will also feel inspired, whatever your situation.

Key Points

- The challenges that face people with type 2 diabetes who are overweight or obese are not necessarily the same as those that people with type 1 diabetes must face. For people who have type 2 diabetes and are overweight or obese, lifestyle modification is a major challenge. It is not easy to lose weight and maintain weight loss indefinitely. It requires a lot of motivation and determination.
- Our patient's stories, and those of many others that we share in this book, continue to inspire us and we have found sharing their stories in turn inspires many others. We hope you also find them inspirational!

2

THE HISTORY OF DIABETES

The greatest joy in life is to accomplish. It is the getting, not the having. It is the giving, not the keeping.

— Sir Frederick Grant Banting

Diabetes has afflicted humans for thousands of years. Before the discovery of insulin by Frederick Banting and Charles Best in the 20th century, type 1 diabetes was a death sentence, leading to death within weeks. The only treatment for someone diagnosed with type 1 diabetes was a starvation diet with very low carbohydrate intake (i.e., a ketogenic diet) and the prognosis was abysmal. Death usually occurred within 6 months of diagnosis. But, like many scientific discoveries, the understanding of diabetes evolved from older observations and knowledge.

Early Physiological Research

The Egyptians described a disease resembling diabetes in manuscripts dating to around 1550 BC. In India, Sushruta (600–500 BC) wrote about a disease he termed *Madhumeha* referring to the sweetness of urine. The physicians of that time diagnosed the condition by seeing if an individual's urine attracted ants. They also noted the extreme thirst and occasional foul breath in patients afflicted with this condition, likely from ketosis, the presence of ketones in the blood and breath due to a lack of carbohydrates. In 250 BC either Apollonius of Memphis or Arateus of Cappadocia coined the term *diabetes* (Greek for "siphon," as patients appeared to pass urine like a siphon).

In 1675 AD a British doctor Thomas Willis coined the term *diabetes mellitus*, the latter a Latin term meaning sweet like honey. It was initially thought to be a disorder of the kidneys or a blood condition. Almost one and a half centuries later, in 1815, chemist Michel Eugène

Chevreul in Paris proved that the cause of the sweetness was, in fact, glucose. In 1848, another chemist, German Hermann von Fehling, developed a quantitative test for measuring glucose in the urine.

Claude Bernard (1813–1878) was a prolific scientist and physiologist, reportedly referred to by the legendary Louis Pasteur as "physiology Itself." He performed an experiment in which he ligated (tied off) the pancreatic ducts of dogs and noted that this led to atrophy of the gland. This set the stage for future studies. William Prout (1785–1850) was the first to describe severe hyperglycemia (high glucose) which led to diabetic coma.

In 1889, Oskar Minkowski and Joseph von Mering were the first two investigators to discover that removal of the pancreas in dogs led to excessive urination (polyuria) and that the urine contained large amounts of glucose. Minkowski was persistent and did an additional experiment in which he implanted a small portion of the removed pancreas underneath the dog's skin. He observed that doing this prevented the high blood glucose. When the implant was removed or once it had spontaneously degenerated, the diabetes returned. This proved that the pancreas was key to regulating blood glucose.

The MacLeod Lab and the Discovery of Insulin

Frederick Banting was an orthopedic surgeon. He had an idea. He approached John MacLeod, a Professor of Physiology at the University of Toronto, requesting laboratory space, a small number of dogs and an assistant in order to perform some novel experiments over an 8-week period in the summer of 1921. Macleod sent Banting two of his students who had just graduated from the physiology and biochemistry course at the University of Toronto - Charles Best and E. Clark Noble.

Banting needed only one assistant and so they flipped a coin to see who would start first. Best won the toss and eagerly joined Banting. Noble was supposed to have replaced Best in July, but before then they came to an understanding that Best would work in the laboratory until the end of the summer. In part, this was due to Best having become very experienced in the surgical techniques required for the experiments. According to some stories, Noble went on a vacation to Europe. In fact, Macleod also went on a vacation - he went off to Scotland and left

Banting and Best to work on their experiments.

Charles Best and Frederick Banting, 1922

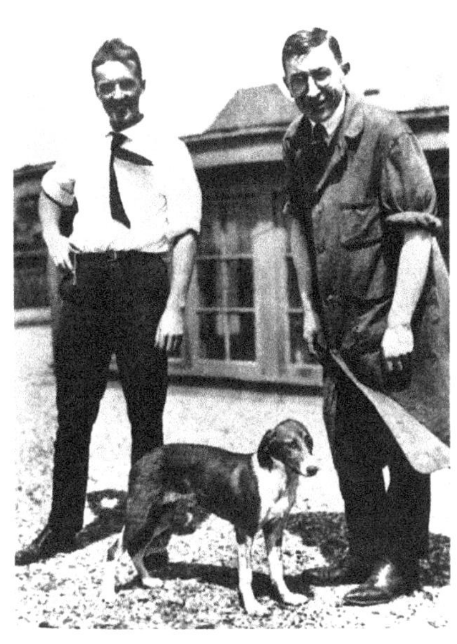

Charles Best (left), Frederick Banting and Marjorie the dog on the roof of the University of Toronto's Medical Building. Reproduced with permission from the Thomas Fisher Rare Book Library, University of Toronto.

Beginning the experiments in May 1921, they harvested pancreatic tissue from dogs, ground it up in a mortar and injected it as an extract into dogs whose pancreases had been removed to render them diabetic. The initial results were not promising, but at the end of July they witnessed success! Injection of the pancreatic extract into one of the dogs lowered the blood glucose and the dog's condition improved. Subsequent injections showed similar results. Banting and Best published and presented their groundbreaking findings in the fall of 1921.

In late 1921, a biochemist James Collip joined the team. He was awarded a Rockefeller scholarship, took a sabbatical from his faculty position at the University of Edmonton and joined the Macleod laboratory. Best continued to work on the production of a pure pancreatic extract for administration to humans.

On January 11th, 1922, a historic experiment was conducted. The pancreatic extract was injected into Leonard Thompson, a 14-year-old boy with type 1 diabetes at Toronto General Hospital. The injection lowered the glucose but had minimal clinical effect, and Thompson developed an abscess at the injection site. Collip was then successful in preparing a purified pancreatic extract, which would pave the way for successful clinical trials and the future of this miraculous drug was assured.

Twelve days after his first injection, Thompson received a second injection of the extract. His blood sugar fell dramatically from 520 to

Leonard Thompson and Patient "J.L."

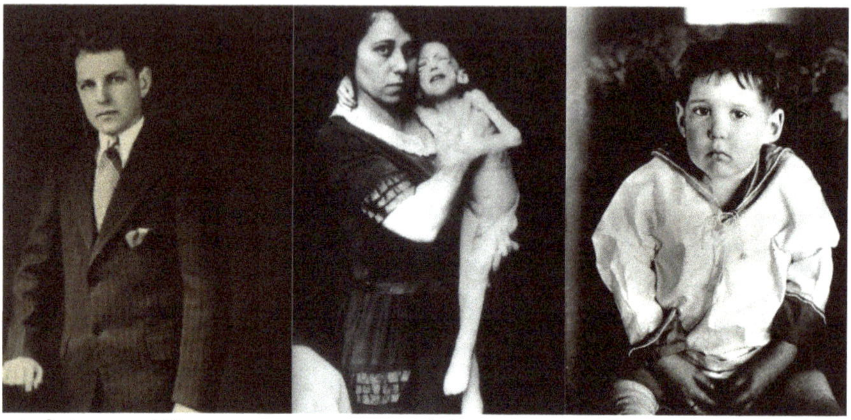

Left: Leonard Thompson, as a young adult some years after commencing the first successful insulin treatment on January 23, 1922, at the age of 14. Having had an allergic reaction to the first injection on January 11 - thought to be due to impurities in the product - eleven days later he received a more purified product, which lowered his blood glucose dramatically. Thompson lived for another 13 years before dying of pneumonia. Middle and right: Patient "J.L." before insulin on December 7, 1922 (15 pounds) and after insulin on February 26, 1923 (30 pounds). Photo courtesy of Eli Lilly and Company Archives.

120 mg/dL and ketones disappeared from the urine. He received further regular injections and lived for 13 more years (unprecedented longevity for someone with type 1 diabetes at that time) before succumbing to pneumonia.

Banting and MacLeod received the Nobel Prize in Physiology or Medicine in 1923. Banting was incensed that Best was not a recipient and shared his monetary winnings with him. Macleod subsequently shared his prize money with Collip.

After the Discovery

Charles Best started medical school in the Fall of 1922 while remaining director of the Connaught Laboratories where insulin was being produced. He graduated first in his class and went on to become a Professor of Physiology at the University of Toronto, succeeding James Macleod. He died in 1978 at the age of 79. He and James Collip sold the patent for what was now known as insulin to the University of Toronto for a mere one dollar! They never wanted to personally profit from it and wanted every patient with diabetes to be able to afford this life saving medicine. Banting had refused to have his name on the patent - he felt it was unethical for doctors to profit from a discovery that would save lives.

Following the discovery of insulin, Banting was elected to the new Banting and Best Chair of Medical Research, which was gifted by the Legislature of the Province of Ontario. His research interests were remarkably diverse, and they ranged from cancer and silicosis to mechanisms of drowning.

Just before the start of the Second World War, Banting took an interest in aviation medicine. This resulted in his participation in research concerning the physiological changes that occur in pilots operating high altitude combat aircraft. He also was involved in research that focused on treating mustard gas burns incurred by soldiers during the war. Astoundingly, Banting even exposed himself to the gas and potential antidotes to test their efficacy! Sadly, Banting died in a plane crash in 1941, at the age of 49.

James Collip returned to the University of Edmonton, where he became head of a new department of biochemistry and spent his career researching hormones. His career thrived and he was appointed as Dean of Medicine at the University of Western Ontario.

Macleod continued research on insulin in fish and then returned to Scotland in 1928 to become Regius Professor of Physiology at Aberdeen University and later Dean of the University of Aberdeen Medical Faculty.

Macleod did not continue to work on insulin, but he remained an active researcher, lecturer and author. In his spare time, he pursued his passions of golf, motorcycling and painting. He was married to Mary W. McWalter, but they never had children. He died in 1935 in Aberdeen at the age of 58 years.

The Insulin Story Continues

After the discovery of insulin, scientists initially worked to obtain purer preparations of insulin that caused fewer allergic reactions. Efforts then focused on how to extend insulin's duration of action, since the initial preparations only produced an effect for about six hours.

In the late 1930s, scientists discovered that by combining the insulin with a protein called protamine, they could extend the duration of action of the insulin by slowing its absorption into the blood after it was injected. This was followed by the development of a zinc-protamine preparation that could lower blood glucose levels for over 24 hours. The types of insulin currently used are discussed in chapter 16 on page 131.

It was not until 1955, however, that the actual composition of insulin in terms of its amino acids (the building blocks of proteins) was discovered by the British biochemist Frederick Sanger. He received the Nobel Prize for this seminal work. Another scientist, Dorothy Crowfoot Hodgkin, subsequently received the Nobel Prize in 1964 for her work describing the structure of insulin.

The next chapter in the insulin story was research about how to measure it in the blood. This was achieved in 1961 by Drs. Solomon Berson and Rosalyn Yallow. They used a method called radioimmunoassay, whereby radioactive antibodies – the specifically-targeted "arrows" of the immune system – are used to target and count blood proteins such as hormones. Their developments paved the way for the measurement of many more proteins and hormones. Dr. Yallow was awarded the Nobel Prize in Physiology or Medicine in 1977 for her outstanding scientific contributions.

The ability to measure insulin in the blood paved the way for advances in our understanding of how insulin affects glucose, protein and fat metabolism, the causes and natural history of diabetes and its treatment. Over the century, since the discovery of insulin, many noteworthy advances have been made in our understanding of who is at risk for developing diabetes, the causes of the different types of diabetes, as well as major advances in the comprehensive treatment of diabetes. We have aimed to cover all these aspects in this book, including the evolution of insulin treatments, summarized in a figure on page 133.

Key Points

- In 1675 AD, a British doctor Thomas Willis coined the term diabetes mellitus, the latter a Latin term meaning sweet like honey.
- Twelve days after his first injection, Leonard Thompson received a second injection of pancreas extract. His blood sugar fell dramatically from 520 to 120 mg/dL and ketones in the urine disappeared. He received further treatments and lived for 13 more years, before dying of pneumonia.
- Banting and MacLeod received the Nobel Prize in Physiology or Medicine in 1923.
- Banting was incensed that Best was not a recipient and shared his monetary winnings with him. Macleod subsequently shared his prize money with Collip.

3

DIABETES: A PRIMER

I have high blood sugars, and type 2 diabetes is not going to kill me. But I just have to eat right, and exercise, and lose weight, and watch what I eat, and I will be fine for the rest of my life.

—Tom Hanks

Diabetes is the commonest metabolic disorder known to affect humans. There are currently more than 460 million people in the world with diabetes, and this number is expected to grow to 700 million by 2045. Prediabetes, the precursor of diabetes, afflicts a similar number of individuals worldwide. Hence the number of people with diabetes and prediabetes exceeds 1 billion.

In the United States there are over 30 million people with diabetes, 95% of whom have type 2 diabetes. It is estimated that the number of people with diabetes in the United States will exceed 50 million in the next 20 to 25 years. At present, the number of people in the United States with prediabetes exceeds 80 million.

Diabetes is rampant in many different parts of the world. In some parts of the Middle East, such as Saudi Arabia, approximately 25% of adults have type 2 diabetes. In multiple countries throughout the world the prevalence of diabetes in adults exceeds 10% of the population. A very thorough and detailed picture of diabetes has been published by the International Diabetes Federation. Impressively, it is available in multiple languages, including Arabic, Chinese, English, French, Korean, Russian and Spanish.

As you will observe in subsequent chapters, diabetes can affect many different organs in the body. The healthcare costs related to the management of diabetes and its complications add up to astounding figures. The annual expenditure worldwide in 2019 was estimated to bc $760 billion and is projected to skyrocket to $845 billion by 2045.

But, as you will see throughout this book, there is a lot that can be done by people who are at risk for or who have diabetes to reduce these costs - by preventing or controlling their diabetes, and even getting their diabetes into remission. In so doing, many of the complications that impact so much on quality and cost of life can be prevented.

Normal Physiology of Glucose Control

Mrs. C, a 42-year-old Hispanic woman, has a "healthy" breakfast consisting of two eggs, two slices of whole grain toast, a cup of coffee and some blueberries. She does not have diabetes. Let's examine how her blood glucose levels remain within the normal range, despite ingesting significant amounts of carbohydrate.

After swallowing, her food is digested by enzymes in the gastrointestinal tract. The carbohydrates are absorbed into the bloodstream as glucose. The rising glucose levels cause the pancreatic beta cells to secrete insulin, which then stimulates cells in other organs

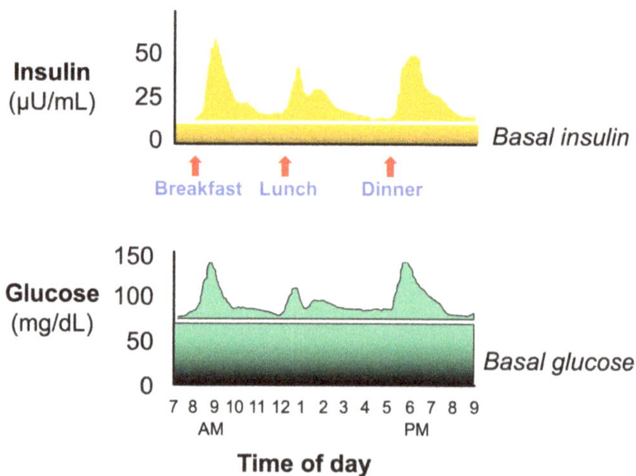

The normal physiology of insulin secretion in response to food ingestion. The beta cells of the pancreas always secrete some insulin - this is called basal insulin secretion. When food is eaten, and glucose levels start rising there is a rapid rise in insulin secretion to ensure that glucose levels do not rise too high. Once the glucose levels start returning to normal, insulin secretion returns to basal levels.

of the body to absorb glucose, where it is used for energy production. As the glucose levels in the blood decrease to the baseline level, the secretion of insulin also decreases proportionally so that the blood glucose levels gradually drop into the normal range, but – importantly – that they do not drop too low! For someone who is fasting, their blood glucose does not drop to dangerously low levels because the liver is able to produce enough glucose from other energy stores – a phenomenon known as **gluconeogenesis** ("new production of glucose").

This is the normal yet elegant physiology in which the pancreas and liver play a central role in regulating glucose levels.

How Do We Define and Diagnose Diabetes?

A normal glucose level when someone has been fasting (a "fasting glucose") is less than 100 mg/dL (5.6 mmol/L). And two hours after a meal or a **glucose tolerance test**, the normal value is less than 140 mg/dL (7.8 mmol/L). Another test that measures glucose levels, but usefully reflects average levels over a period of months, is Hemoglobin A1c (HbA1c), the amount of glucose bound to the oxygen-carrying hemoglobin protein in red blood cells (glucose has a slight tendency to bind to proteins over time). A normal HbA1c is less than 5.7%.

The **glucose tolerance test** (GTT) is a test for how well your body metabolizes sugar. E.g., after 8 hours of fasting, a patient is given 8 ounces (237 milliliters) of a syrupy glucose solution with 2.6 ounces (75 grams) of sugar. Their blood glucose is measured 2 hours later.

Diabetes

Diabetes is diagnosed when the:

- fasting glucose is 126 mg/dL or higher (7 mmol/L); or
- glucose level two hours after a meal or a glucose tolerance test is 200 mg/dL or higher (11.1 mmol/L); or
- HbA1c is 6.5% or higher.

We usually require two abnormal values on two separate occasions to confirm the diagnosis.

Prediabetes

Given the numbers above, you may be wondering how we define people who have a fasting glucose between 101 and 126 mg/dL, or a

The Criteria for Diagnosing Metabolic Syndrome

Test	Criterion
Waist circumference	35 inches (89 cm) – women >40 inches (102 cm) – men
Blood pressure	130/85 mm Hg or higher
Fasting blood glucose	100 mg/dL (5.6 mmol/l) or higher
Fasting triglycerides	150 mg/dL or higher
Fasting HDL cholesterol ("good" cholesterol)	<40 mg/dL (1.04 mmol/l) in men <50 mg/dL (1.3 mmol/l) in women

random glucose between 140 and 200 mg/dL, or whose HbA1c is between 5.7 and 6.5%. We refer to individuals in this category as having **prediabetes**.

The prediabetes category is important because it identifies people who are at risk for the development of diabetes. More importantly, people with prediabetes often have other components of **metabolic syndrome** – a group of clinical signs associated with an increased risk for atherosclerotic cardiovascular disease, and therefore stroke, heart attack and peripheral vascular disease (clogged arteries of the legs).

More than 50% of people over the age of 50 in the United States have metabolic syndrome. And there are a staggering 80+ million people with prediabetes – this is almost 35% of the population!

According to a 2021 study published in the *Journal of the American Medical Association* (JAMA), the risk for developing diabetes if you have prediabetes ranges from 15 to 30% over five years. However, older people with prediabetes (average age 75 years) may have a lower risk for progression to diabetes.

Type I and Type 2 Diabetes

There are two main types of diabetes: type I and type 2. What is the difference?

Type 1 diabetes is an autoimmune disorder involving the destruction of the **beta cells of the pancreas**, the cells that produce insulin. “Autoimmune” means that for some reason the body's immune system is attacking its own cells, in this case the pancreatic beta cells. What causes this to occur is unknown. It may be related to exposure to a virus or chemical, and it certainly has some genetic components, but the exact cause remains elusive. We do know that there is some familial predisposition to developing it, but this is not very strong. In fact, a child of a parent with type 1 diabetes has no more than about a 2% chance of developing the same problem.

Type 2 Diabetes

Type 2 diabetes is a completely different disorder. It is the most common form and affects almost 95% of people with diabetes. It is caused by a combination of factors.

Most people with type 2 diabetes have what is called **insulin resistance**. This means that the insulin produced by the beta cells is less effective than in normal people. Insulin's main action is to push glucose into the cells of the body where it is used as the main source

The Two Major Contributing Factors for Developing Type 2 Diabetes

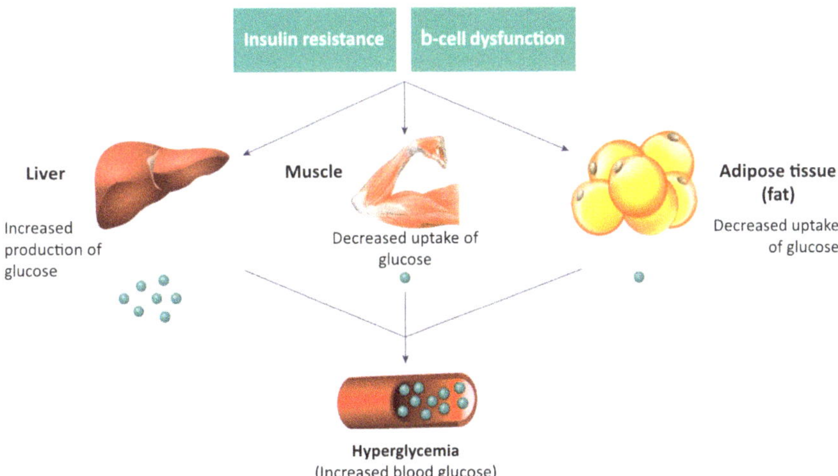

The two major contributing factors for the development of type 2 diabetes: insulin resistance and β-cell dysfunction. Adapted from the ASCEND (Academy for Science and Continuing Education in Diabetes and Obesity) Program. http://www.ASCEND-diabetes-obesity.com.

of energy. Insulin resistance usually occurs many years before the actual development of diabetes. The reason why people don't develop diabetes when they become insulin resistant is because the beta cells are initially able to compensate for this resistance by making more insulin. However, over time the beta cells begin to fail in their ability to make as much insulin, and as they produce less insulin, so the glucose levels tend to rise, leading initially to prediabetes and then ultimately to overt diabetes.

Hence there are two major issues at play in people who develop type 2 diabetes: insulin resistance and dysfunction of the pancreatic beta cells. Insulin resistance is more common in overweight or obese individuals. Most people who develop type 2 diabetes are indeed overweight or obese – roughly 90% of people with type 2 diabetes fall into this category. As people gain more weight so the insulin resistance increases, and this is compounded by a sedentary lifestyle. We will discuss this in more detail later in the book.

There is a greater familial predisposition to type 2 diabetes than type 1 diabetes. Indeed, in a study of identical twins, it was found that if one twin had type 2 diabetes there was a 90% chance that the other had it or would also develop it. We do not know the exact nature of the genes that are responsible for the development of type 2 diabetes but there is clearly a greater genetic predisposition to develop this form of diabetes than type I. However, environmental factors that lead to being overweight or obese play a major role in the development of this form of diabetes.

Other Forms of Diabetes

There are other rare, genetic forms of diabetes that are usually only diagnosed by a diabetologist. Clinically, the presentation is similar to that of someone who has type 2 diabetes. However, individuals with these forms present with a strong family history of diabetes and are not usually overweight or obese.

There is one other important form of diabetes that needs to be mentioned and that is **gestational diabetes**. This is defined as the development of diabetes during pregnancy. During normal pregnancy, the placenta makes certain growth factors that cross into the maternal circulation and cause insulin resistance. Gestational diabetes is common, and effects up to 10% of all pregnancies. It usually resolves following the pregnancy, but women who develop gestational diabetes have a significantly greater risk of developing type 2 diabetes later in life. We discuss gestational diabetes in a separate chapter (see page 191).

Should You Be Screened for Diabetes?

The American Diabetes Association recommends that everyone aged 45 or older be screened for diabetes. The screening test is a simple blood test that measures either **HbA1c** (see page 140), a **fasting glucose** or a **random** (non-fasting state) **glucose**.

The HbA1c does not need to be measured in the fasting state as it reflects average glucose concentrations over the preceding three months. This makes it a very convenient screening test. Any abnormal result needs to be verified on a second occasion. We will still sometimes perform a glucose tolerance test in individuals who are at risk for diabetes and in whom one of the above tests is equivocal. As stated above, a fasting glucose of 126 mg/dL or greater, or a glucose two hours after the sugary drink of 200 mg/dL or more, is diagnostic of diabetes.

> Sometimes the diagnosis of diabetes is first made incidentally, for example, when a patient is admitted to the hospital with a major illness such as pneumonia, a heart attack, or following major trauma.

It is recommended that people who have risk factors for diabetes be screened before the age of 45, if they are overweight or obese and have at least one additional risk factor for diabetes:

- A first degree relative with diabetes.
- Hypertension (high blood pressure).
- Hyperlipidemia (high blood lipids).
- Women with polycystic ovarian syndrome.
- A history of gestational diabetes.
- A history of cardiovascular disease (i.e., coronary artery disease – e.g., angina or history of prior heart attack).
- Certain ethnic populations e.g., African American, Hispanic, Asian American, or Native American people.

In August 2021, the United States Preventative Task Force revised its

Major Differences Between Type 1 and Type 2 Diabetes

	Type 1 diabetes	Type 2 diabetes
Percent of total incidence of diabetes	5	95
Age of onset	Mostly in childhood, adolescence and young adult, but may occur at any age	Usually adults over 40; increasingly in younger people including children
Major contributing cause	Autoimmune disease destroys insulin-producing cells of the pancreas	Insulin resistance and decreased insulin secretion
Typical symptoms at presentation	The "classic presentation" includes excessive thirst, urination, weight loss, blurred vision	Often none but may develop "classic symptoms" if glucose levels are very high
Risk for complications	Similar in both: related to disease duration and degree of control	
Pharmacological treatment	Insulin is essential	Can be managed with a variety of medications other than insulin, but insulin may be required

recommendation that screening for prediabetes and type 2 diabetes begin at age 35 for those who have risk factors for the disease. If the screening test is normal, then it should be repeated at a minimum of every three years. For people who have prediabetes, screening should be repeated annually.

What Are the Symptoms of Diabetes?

People with type 1 diabetes often present with classical symptoms, including thirst, excessive urination, blurred vision, loss of weight, fatigue or recurrent urinary or genital infections or other infections. In some cases, people present much more severely, with symptoms indicating **ketoacidosis**, the presence of high levels of acidic ketones in the blood due to the body's "carbohydrate-starved" state. The symptoms of ketoacidosis include extreme thirst, nausea, vomiting, abdominal pain, and somnolence. It is a serious situation as, if left untreated, it can progress to coma and even death.

Ketoacidosis occurs when there is very little insulin present, which leads to a massive accumulation of glucose in the blood. But with a severe lack of insulin, glucose is not able to get into the cells, where it is essential for energy. And so instead, the liver starts producing ketones, using fatty acids (the building blocks of fat) as an alternative source of energy for cells. However, these ketones are acidic and accumulate in the blood. This is a serious condition and needs to be treated urgently.

Many people with type 2 diabetes have no symptoms, hence the need for screening. In the United States, it is estimated that 25% of people with type 2 diabetes are walking around unaware that they have the disease. In other parts of the world this number is even higher - 50% of people are undiagnosed!

The classical symptoms usually occur when glucose levels are high. Indeed, the higher the glucose level the greater the likelihood of symptoms occurring. Mild elevations in glucose are often not associated with symptoms (i.e., asymptomatic) which is why screening is so important.

Sometimes the diagnosis of diabetes is first made incidentally, for example, when a patient is admitted to the hospital with a major illness such as pneumonia, a heart attack, or following major trauma.

The Complications of Diabetes

The complications of diabetes include chronic damage to large blood vessels (**macrovascular disease**), leading to increased risk of heart disease, stroke and peripheral vascular disease; and chronic damage to small vessels (**microvascular disease**), leading to visual loss (**retinopathy**), renal failure (**nephropathy**) and nerve damage (**neuropathy**). Each of these are discussed in detail in subsequent chapters.

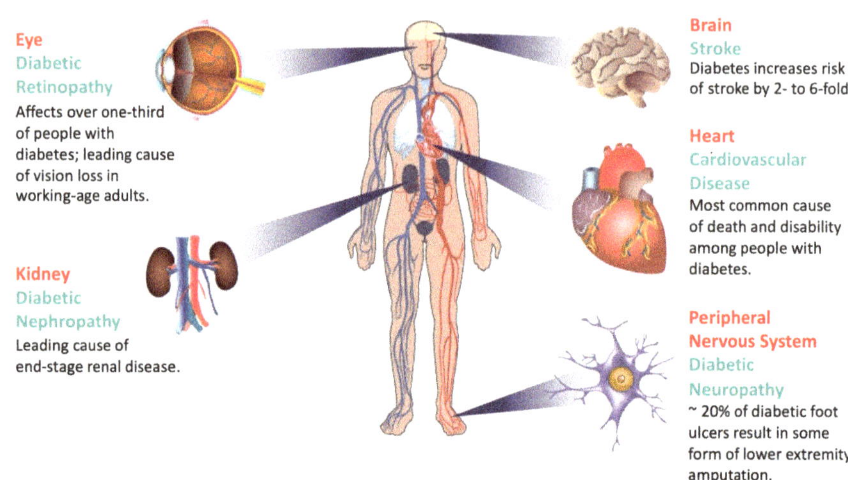

The major complications of both type 1 and type 2 diabetes. Adapted from the ASCEND (Academy for Science and Continuing Education in Diabetes and Obesity) Program. http://www.ASCEND-diabetes-obesity.com.

Key Points

- Type 1 diabetes is an autoimmune disorder that is characterized by destruction of the beta cells of the pancreas, the cells that produce insulin. Autoimmune means that for some reason the body's immune system is attacking its own cells, in this case the beta cells.
- Type 2 diabetes is a completely different disorder. It is the most common form and affects almost 95% of people with diabetes. It is caused by a combination of factors and the two major issues are insulin resistance and dysfunction of the pancreatic beta cells.
- Many people with type 2 diabetes have no symptoms, hence the need for screening. In the United States, it is estimated that 25% of people with type 2 diabetes are walking around unaware that they have the disease. In other parts of the world this number is even higher - 50% of people are undiagnosed!
- The complications of diabetes include chronic damage to large blood vessels (macrovascular disease), leading to increased risk of heart disease, stroke and peripheral vascular disease, and small vessels (microvascular disease), leading to visual loss (retinopathy), renal failure (nephropathy) and nerve damage (neuropathy).

4

THE PREVENTION OF DIABETES

An ounce of prevention is worth a pound of cure.

—Benjamin Franklin

I prevent type 2 diabetes so I can keep traveling, taking pictures, and enjoying my family for the rest of my life.

—Suzi Gomez, 53, participant in the CDC's National Diabetes Prevention Program

Type 2 diabetes can be prevented. Even individuals who have prediabetes, which significantly increases their risk for developing diabetes, can prevent progression to overt diabetes. The most effective way is through lifestyle modification: weight loss through diet, and exercise. This is supported by three large clinical trials conducted in different parts of the world.

The Evidence

In the United States, a study called the Diabetes Prevention Program demonstrated that after three years of lifestyle modification resulting in weight loss of 7% body weight, there was a staggering 58% reduction in the risk for developing diabetes in people who had prediabetes. The lifestyle modification program included a low-fat diet and regular exercise program comprising 150 minutes of moderate intensity exercise, such as brisk walking, per week.

In a similar study conducted in Finland the same results were obtained. And a third study conducted in China, called the Da Qing study, showed that lifestyle modification significantly improved outcomes compared to the control group, who did not participate in any specific "program."

The people who took part in these studies were followed up for a number of years after the study had been concluded. The longest follow-up data comes from the Da Qing study and is very impressive! *Thirty years* after the study ended, the researchers reported that the people who had been in the initial lifestyle modification arm of the study *still* had a 39% reduction in risk for the development of diabetes, even though not everyone had continued to adhere to the lifestyle modifications that they had during the trial. Furthermore, they had lower overall mortality rates, including cardiovascular mortality! The US and Finnish studies have also shown that, even after 10 to 15 years, the lifestyle interventions substantially reduce the risk for progression to type 2 diabetes. So, there appears to be an impressive lasting positive effect when people eat healthier and exercise regularly, which we call a "legacy effect."

> Multiple large long-term studies from across the world have shown that lifestyle interventions (i.e., good diet and regular exercise) continue to have a significant benefit on cardiovascular health and longevity, even years after they have stopped. This "legacy effect" is strong evidence for the power of diet and exercise!

Can Medications Prevent Diabetes?

Metformin was studied in the Diabetes Prevention Program. There was a 30% reduction in risk for developing diabetes in those people taking metformin. The individuals who did best were those who had a BMI of >35, those under 60 years of age and women who had a previous history of gestational diabetes.

> We use the **body mass index** (BMI) to determine weight status. It is calculated as weight in kg divided by height (height in m²). The optimal BMI is 19–24.9 kg/m². 25 or more is considered overweight, and obesity is defined as 30 or more.

Other medications that we use to treat diabetes have also been studied for the prevention of diabetes. These include medications that delay the absorption of glucose from the bowel (alpha-glucosidase inhibitors), thiazolidinediones, and glucagon-like peptide-1 (GLP-1) receptor agonists. The reduction in risk for the development of diabetes with these medications ranges from 25% to 60%.

None of these medications have been officially approved for the prevention of diabetes by the US Federal Drug Administration (FDA).

Strategies To Prevent Type 2 Diabetes

Strategy	Results
1. Diet & exercise	Up to 58% risk reduction
2. Medications	
a. Metformin	31% risk reduction
b. Acarbose	25% risk reduction
c. Rosiglitazone*	60% risk reduction
3. Coffee	30% (women) to 54% (men) risk reduction with 6 or more cups of regular or decaffeinated coffee per day

Strategies to prevent type 2 diabetes. * Rosiglitazone use is associated with weight gain and risk of bone fractures, and is not recommended for prevention.

Metformin is the most established, but even this is less effective than lifestyle modification.

We strongly recommend that individuals with prediabetes follow a lifestyle modification program with goals of weight loss and which include regular exercise. This is the most effective way to prevent type 2 diabetes. We also strongly suggest that people who have prediabetes be screened annually for diabetes (for screening methods see page 19).

Preventing Type 1 Diabetes

Interventions to prevent type 1 diabetes are difficult. As you know, type 1 diabetes is caused by a completely different process from type 2 diabetes. It is an autoimmune disease in which the body produces antibodies that attack the insulin-producing beta cells of the pancreas. We know from elegant research done by the late George Eisenbarth when he was at the Joslin Diabetes Center in Boston in the 1980s that these antibodies are present in the blood many years before people develop overt diabetes. In theory, eliminating these antibodies before they have destroyed all the beta cells could prevent progression to diabetes. In practice, this is difficult since it would require some form of immunosuppression (such as the medications that are used in people who have had organ transplants) and these medications have potentially negative side effects.

There is some hope, however. In 2020, scientists published a paper in the *New England Journal of Medicine* showing that teplizumab, a medication that targets certain white blood cells involved in the autoimmune destruction of beta cells, reduced the rate of progression to overt diabetes in people who had these anti-beta cell antibodies present in the blood. This was a relatively short-term study (a "phase 2 study") designed to assess efficacy and safety), but nonetheless it has provided a lot of promise. Longer-term phase 3 studies are currently being conducted.

And What About Coffee?

Many observational studies, conducted in various parts of the world, including the United States, Europe and Asia, have shown that people who drink coffee regularly reduce their risk for the development of type 2 diabetes (see page 35). One of the studies, conducted by researchers at the Harvard School of Public Health, showed a direct relationship between the amount of coffee consumed and the risk for diabetes, with the risk being cut by up to 50% for people drinking ten cups of coffee per day. The risk reduction was also shown for people who drank decaffeinated coffee, although it was a bit less than that found in the caffeine drinkers!

Patient Stories: A Diagnosis of Prediabetes

PD was 32 years old when she was first seen. Of Hispanic heritage, she was single and worked as an associate at a major law firm in Boston. She was in good health, although she had gained 24 pounds [11 kg] in the past five years, which she attributed to her busy work schedule interfering with her time to exercise and cook her own food regularly. She took no medications. She was 5'4" tall, weighed 162 pounds [73.5 kg], and hence her BMI was 28 kg/m^2, which is considered to be overweight. She did not drink alcohol or smoke.

Other than feeling somewhat fatigued (likely related to long work hours) she had no symptoms. Her father was diagnosed with type 2 diabetes when he was 52. He was overweight, and she was concerned that she was "heading" to a similar fate.

Her physical examination was normal, as was her blood pressure.

Her primary care clinician had done the appropriate screening tests and had forwarded them. They showed that routine blood tests, including liver function and kidney function tests were normal. However, her fasting glucose was 109 mg/dL (6 mmol/L) and HbA1c was 6.0% both of which are diagnostic of prediabetes.

PD wondered what the best plan of action would be for her to reduce her risk for developing type 2 diabetes. She had heard that metformin might be a good medication to take.

Our advice at this point: We encouraged her to modify her lifestyle as the primary strategy to prevent diabetes, based on the scientific evidence in the medical literature. The key components of treatment included diet modification and regular exercise (at least 150 minutes of moderate intensity exercise per week). The goal was for her to lose at least 7% of her body weight (i.e., approximately 11 pounds [5 kg]). Fortunately, she was very motivated and said she would see a nutritionist and get a personal trainer, which she did. She elected to follow a relatively low-carbohydrate diet and eliminated many starchy foods.

She was seen in follow-up three months later and had lost six pounds and was working out 35 to 40 minutes a day, five times a week doing a combination of aerobic and strength training exercises. Six months later she had lost an additional five pounds. Her fasting blood glucose was now 98 mg/dL and her HbA1c was 5.6%! She was ecstatic and highly motivated to continue with this course of action.

One year later her primary care physician informed us that she had continued to lose weight and her HbA1c was now 5.3%.

Take-Home Message

People who are motivated and can adhere to dietary modifications and an exercise regimen that leads to weight loss can prevent diabetes developing indefinitely.

Key Points

- Type 2 diabetes can be prevented. The most effective way to prevent type 2 diabetes is through lifestyle modification, i.e., weight loss through diet and exercise.
- The longest follow-up data comes from the Da Qing study in China and is very impressive: the researchers reported that the people in the initial lifestyle modification arm of the study had a 39% reduction in risk for the development of diabetes. Furthermore, they had lower overall mortality rates, including cardiovascular mortality!

5

COFFEE AND DIABETES

Coffee is a superfood!

—Sanjiv Chopra, MD

Coffee is the number one beverage consumed in the world. 2.25 billion cups of coffee are consumed every day! Is this good or bad?

The Protective Effect of Coffee

Researchers from Brigham and Women's Hospital and the Harvard School of Public Health conducted an 18-year study that started in 1980. They tracked 125,000 individuals and reported the results in the *Annals of Internal Medicine* in 2004. Men and women who drank 6 or more cups of coffee daily - regular or decaffeinated - reduced their risk of developing Type 2 Diabetes by 54% and 30% respectively.

A study published in the *Archives of Internal Medicine* in 2009 validated these 2004 findings. The authors examined 18 studies involving 450,000 participants - this is referred to as a meta-analysis. They concluded that with every additional cup of coffee consumed, there was a 7% reduction in the excess risk of developing diabetes. Both studies demonstrated that the more coffee one consumed, the greater the reduction in risk of developing diabetes, and that the protective effect with decaffeinated coffee was less robust.

In another interesting Harvard study published in the journal *Diabetologia* in 2014, researchers examined changes in coffee intake in three cohorts of men and women. They followed 95,974 women and 27,759 men and assessed the data every four years. The conclusions are again quite striking. Increased coffee consumption was associated with a lower risk of developing type 2 diabetes, while decreased coffee consumption was linked to a higher risk of developing type 2 diabetes.

It is worth noting that changes in tea consumption had no effect on risk of developing type 2 diabetes.

Coffee's salubrious effect is hypothesized to be due to one or more ingredients. It is rich in chlorogenic acid and tocopherols, both powerful antioxidants, as well as minerals such as magnesium. All of these have been shown to favorably affect glucose metabolism by improving insulin sensitivity.

Voltaire, the French Philosopher, died in 1778 at the ripe old age of 83 and is purported to have enjoyed between 50 and 72 cups of coffee each day!

Coffee and the Microbiome

More recently, coffee has been shown to alter the gut **microbiome** (see chapter 6, page 41). There are 100 trillion bacteria in our gastrointestinal (GI) tract, and around 1000 different species. This massive and dynamic collection of organisms and their DNA has even been called the "Second Human Genome" and the "Inner Bacterial Rainforest," and might also be considered a newly discovered organ. The type and number of different bacteria is affected by the way we are born - either via vaginal delivery or by c-section, where we live, whether we received antibiotics in early childhood, certain medications that we take (for example, proton pump inhibitors usually prescribed for severe heartburn), what we eat (e.g., non-vegetarian or vegan diet) and what we drink, including coffee!

The composition of the microbiome has implications in obesity, diabetes, cancer, arthritis, liver disease, mental health and even perhaps in autism. It is currently one of the hottest topics of investigation in medicine.

In a small study of 34 participants, researchers from Baylor College of Medicine presented their findings at the Annual Meeting of the American College of Gastroenterology in 2019. They found that the microbiome of coffee drinkers had an abundance of two bacterial genera - *Fecalibacterium* and *Roseburia* - while having low levels of *Erysipelatoclostridium*, which is considered a potentially harmful bacterial genus. This was postulated to be the mechanism whereby coffee exerted favorable effects.

Other Health Benefits

Even if you have type 2 diabetes, consuming 3 to 4 cups of regular or decaffeinated coffee per day lowers cardiovascular mortality by almost 25%!

Coffee drinkers also have a lower risk of:

- **Cirrhosis** of the liver: There is a dose dependent effect in that there is a greater reduction in people who drink 4 cups of coffee per day compared to those who drink 2 cups.
- Seven common **cancers**:
    1. Primary cancer of the liver (the third most frequent cause of cancer mortality in the world and in 11 countries such as Egypt and Mongolia the number 1 cause of cancer mortality). Drinking 2 cups of regular coffee per day lowers the risk by 40%.
    2. Head and neck cancer.
    3. Breast cancer.
    4. Endometrial (uterine) cancer.
    5. Metastatic prostate cancer.
    6. Colon cancer.
    7. Skin cancer.
- **Gout**.
- **Parkinson's disease** and early cognitive decline (i.e., early Alzheimer's disease).
- **Suicide**.
- **Atrial fibrillation** (a common heart arrhythmia), which, if untreated, can lead to heart failure and stroke. A recent study showed that coffee consumption of 1 to 3 cups per day reduced the risk of atrial fibrillation in men.
- **Mortality**! People with type 2 diabetes who drank coffee were shown in a study published in 2006 in the journal *Diabetologia* to have a significantly lower total and cardiovascular mortality.

Coffee drinking in moderate amounts may also reduce the risk of stroke and limit the deleterious consequences of suffering a stroke.

Side Effects

What about the side effects of coffee?

People who drink coffee may have an increased risk of

Coffee Drinkers Have a Lower Risk of Common Cancers

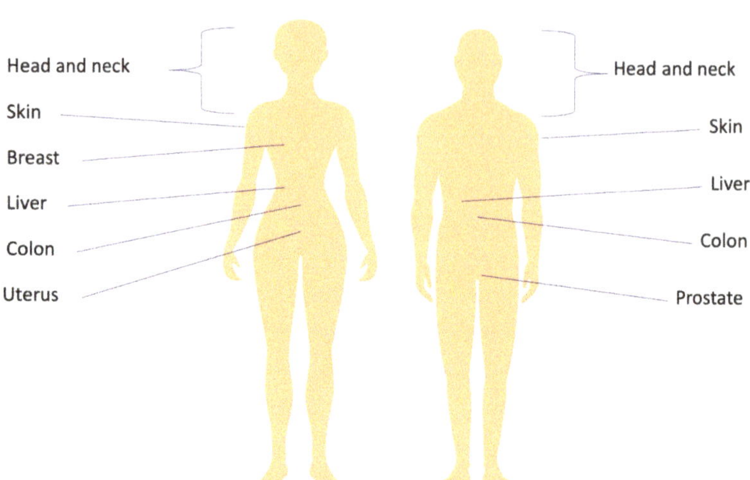

gastroesophageal reflux disease (GERD; heartburn), tremor, insomnia, and minor increases in blood pressure. These effects can be easily countered by commonly used medicines – the beneficial health benefits of coffee far outweigh these relatively minor side effects.

Recent Noteworthy Studies

The "Holy Grail" of evidence would be studies that document that coffee drinkers have lower mortality rates. This is indeed the case! At least half a dozen studies published in prestigious medical journals have shown that coffee drinkers – both men and women – have lower total and cause-specific mortality. The studies revealed that different kinds of coffee preparations have equivalent benefits and that people from different ethnic backgrounds (Caucasian, Asian American, Hispanic) derive the same benefits.

Coffee drinkers have a significantly lower risk of:

- Parkinson's disease.
- Alzheimer's dementia.
- Stroke.
- Atrial fibrillation.
- Cardiovascular mortality.
- Cirrhosis of the liver.
- Diabetes.
- Gout.
- Death from suicide.
- LOWER TOTAL AND CAUSE-SPECIFIC MORTALITY.

Key Points

- Men and women who drank 6 or more cups of coffee daily - regular or decaffeinated - reduced their risk of developing type 2 diabetes by 54% and 30% respectively.
- Even if you have type 2 diabetes, consuming 3 to 4 cups of regular or decaffeinated coffee per day lowers cardiovascular mortality by almost 25%!

6

THE MICROBIOME AND DIABETES

Microbes Maketh Man.

—Cover of *The Economist*,
August 18th, 2012

The microbiome refers to the vast number of bacteria, viruses and fungi that inhabit our body. There are an estimated 100 trillion bacteria in our gut, well over twice the number of human cells! The microbiome has 8 million genes - just compare that to humans, who have only 23,000. No wonder the microbiome has been referred to as the "Second Human Genome," the "Inner Bacterial Rainforest" and a "newly discovered organ" - estimated to weigh 3 pounds [1.36 kg].

It has been a prominent topic in media in the last few years, including a cover story in the *Economist* in 2012, *Time* Magazine and newspapers globally. It continues to be prominently discussed in scientific journals like *Gastroenterology*, the official journal of the American Gastroenterology Association. Since its discovery, many academic institutions have created specialized centers for clinical and basic science research on the microbiome, and garnered collaboration with numerous subspecialty disciplines in medicine.

The microbiome is shaped by whether we were born by natural birth or c-section, whether we had breast milk from our mothers or were bottle fed, whether we received antibiotics during infancy, what kind of foods we consume, where we live, whether we drink coffee, what medicines we take, and whether we exercise, and more!

Our gastrointestinal (GI) tract is sterile at birth, but within a few hours it is colonized by bacteria which establish themselves within a month. More than 1000 species of microbes take up residence in this "house" and embed themselves in a biofilm - a thin layer of microbes coating the interior wall of the GI tract.

The Gut Microbiome and Type 2 Diabetes

In the last five years, there has been an exponential increase in scientific studies addressing the role of the gut microbiome in obesity and type 2 diabetes. It has been postulated that an alteration in gut microbiota plays a seminal role in the development of obesity and type 2 diabetes. Certain gut bacteria produce butyrate, which has beneficial effects on fat and glucose metabolism. Butyrate is a short-chain fatty acid that supports digestive health and helps control inflammation, including a protective effect against colorectal cancer.

What is interesting is that the microbiome in obese individuals has been shown to be *more* effective in harvesting energy from the diet than in individuals without obesity.

An article published by Hartstra and colleagues published in *Diabetes Care* in 2015, "Insights into the role of the microbiome in obesity and type 2 diabetes," summarized the state of knowledge up to that point in time. They point out that products of intestinal microbes such as

The Fabulous Microbiome

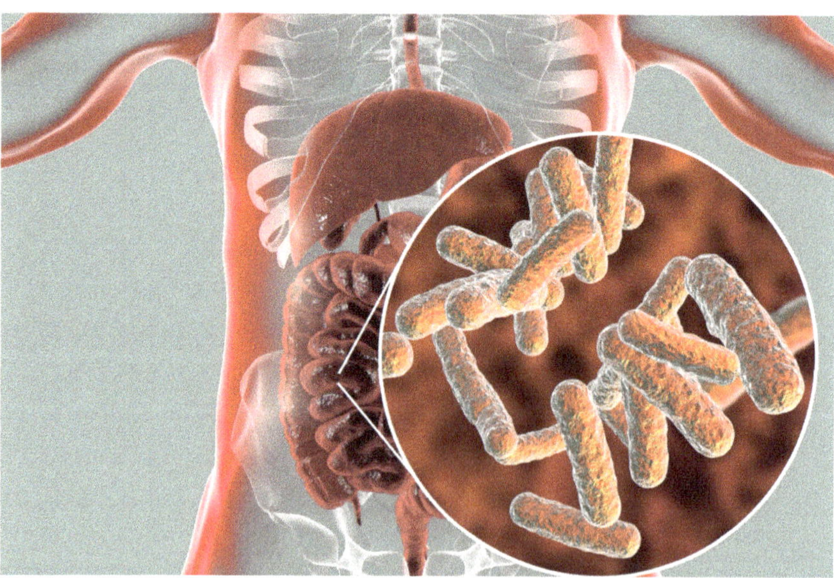

The gut microbiome consists of bacteria that are both health-promoting and potentially harmful. The bacteria can be *anti*-inflammatory or *pro*inflammatory. Exercise and healthy foods, such as fermented products, certain yoghurts and coffee, can favorably affect the gut microbiome.

butyrate may induce beneficial metabolic effects through multiple mechanisms including activation of intestinal gluconeogenesis (glucose production by the cells of the intestine).

Remarkably, after bariatric surgery there is improvement or remission of type 2 diabetes in 50% to 75% of people (see chapter 18, page 163). The weight loss and gut hormonal changes associated with bariatric surgery undoubtedly contribute to these beneficial changes. Astonishingly, however, there are some patients who achieve normal or near normal blood sugar levels within days after surgery, before any significant weight loss has occurred. Studies have shown that the gut microbiome of these patients is already favorably altered.

Zeevi and colleagues published some very interesting and provocative findings in the journal *Cell* in 2015. They studied 800 individuals and their blood sugar responses to a wide variety and number of meals. They found that even after the same food, blood sugar levels were strikingly different amongst individuals, and that this was predicated – not solely but significantly – by the composition of their gut microbiome.

Non-caloric artificial sweeteners are widely used by millions of people, including those with diabetes. Suez and colleagues published a fascinating study in *Nature* in 2014 showing that artificial sweeteners changed the gut microbiota and induced glucose intolerance, i.e., high blood glucose levels. This suggests that artificial sweeteners may have contributed to the obesity and diabetes epidemics that they were invented to counter!

Eat the right foods to have a healthier gut and promote health! A large study published in *Nature Medicine* in 2021 showed that:

- Highly processed foods, added sugars, salt and additives promoted gut microbes associated with worse cardiovascular and metabolic health.
- Consuming juices, sweetened beverages, white bread, and processed meat led to an increase in microbes associated with poor metabolic health.
- Eating vegetables, nuts, eggs and seafood led to an increase in beneficial gut bacteria.

In the not-too-distant future, strategies to ameliorate or reverse type 2 diabetes will likely include ways to favorably alter the composition of the gut microbiome.

The Psychobiome Revolution

Although unrelated to diabetes in a direct way, the "psychobiome revolution" is an exciting new field of research that illustrates the profound importance of the microbiome, in previously unexpected ways.

A small but fascinating study, "Long-term benefit of Microbiota Transfer Therapy in Autism Symptoms and Gut Microbiota," was published in *Scientific Reports* in 2019. The researchers performed a special type of fecal transplant called microbiota transfer therapy (MTT) in people with an autism spectrum disorder (ASD). Two years following treatment, most of the initial improvements in gut symptoms persisted. In addition, parents reported a slow but steady reduction of ASD's psychological symptoms. An independent evaluator found a remarkable 45% reduction in core ASD symptoms involving language, social interaction, and behavior, at two years post-treatment compared to before treatment began.

Similar studies are ongoing to address the efficacy of this novel approach in people with bipolar disorder, schizophrenia, and schizoaffective disorder. People with schizophrenia have a "break from reality," and often experience auditory and visual hallucinations, while those with schizoaffective disorder usually do not have hallucinations.

We highly recommend Scott C. Anderson's book, *The Psychobiotic Revolution*, if you are interested to learn more about this fascinating area.

The current medications used to treat these psychiatric disorders often lead to weight gain, glucose intolerance and diabetes. If this revolutionary approach to treat these disorders is proven to be beneficial in large-scale and well-conducted trials, it might well be a substitute for pharmacological treatments and reduce the risk of these undesirable side effects of treatment.

Future Therapies

Probiotics are live microorganisms that are supposed to confer health benefits when ingested and are taken by millions of individuals worldwide. The global market has been estimated to be worth $60 billion in 2020. At present, they have been shown to be beneficial in only a few conditions, including antibiotic-associated diarrhea and hepatic encephalopathy, a condition of mental status changes ranging from mild confusion to coma secondary to severe liver disease (usually advanced cirrhosis).

In the future, individuals will likely be prescribed probiotics based on an analysis of their gut microbiome. We refer to this as "precision probiotics." There are already companies that perform lab analysis on an individual's stool sample and recommend dietary changes and supplements, including probiotics, to improve health. Their efficacy remains to be determined.

Fruit flies are remarkably similar to mammals in their biochemical pathways and are often used as animal models to research longevity. Synbiotics (probiotics combined with a herbal supplement) fed to fruit flies have been shown to reduce inflammation and increase lifespan by a dramatic 60%!

Prebiotics are selectively fermented products that change the composition and/or activity of the GI tract microflora and may confer health benefits. There is intense interest in studying these, both alone and in combination with probiotics, for their potential health benefits in humans.

A stool transplant may become part of the therapeutic toolkit to treat type 2 diabetes and obesity. These studies are ongoing. What has been established is that stool transplants are effective in treating patients with refractory C. *difficile* colitis and with irritable bowel syndrome (IBS). Not all stool donors are truly healthy – the concept of super stool donors with the most favorable composition of gut bacteria has recently emerged. We refer to them as "Super Poopers"!

> Potential donors for stool transplants are screened by blood tests for viral hepatitis A, B and C; HIV and syphilis; and their stool is examined for parasites and specific bacteria known as *C. difficile*, which can cause inflammation of the colon.

Potential Applications

The many potential clinical applications derived from our understanding of the gut microbiome include the treatment or prevention of:

- Juvenile arthritis.
- Rheumatoid arthritis.
- Obesity.
- Diabetes.
- Alzheimer's disease.
- Parkinson's disease.
- Hepatic encephalopathy (a state varying from minor confusion to coma seen in patients with advanced liver disease).
- Longevity.
- Autism.

Not Just the Gut!

Most microbiome research has focused on the gut microbiome. However, the microbiome also includes microbes resident in the nostrils, mouth, armpits, skin and vagina. Additionally, although researchers have focused on bacteria, what about the viruses and fungi of the microbiome and their potential implications in health and disease? Indeed, the term "fungibiome" has been coined.

In a fascinating TED talk "What's left to explore?" by biologist and explorer Nathan Wolfe, he informs us about "biological dark matter," the poorly understood genetic material in our genome and in "our microorganisms." The latter accounts for 40–50% of the genetic material in the human gut, 20% of the genetic material in the nose, and 1% of genetic material in sterile blood, and may well be an additional domain of life that needs to be further explored and might even give us clues to the mystery of life and death.

Key Points

- We are discovering more and more about how the microbiome - all the microorganisms associated with our bodies - is intricately and essentially involved in nearly every aspect of our health. A personalized "second genome," it is shaped by many factors, including whether we were born by natural birth or c-section, whether we had breast milk from our mothers or were bottle fed, whether we received antibiotics during infancy, what kind of foods we consume, where we live, whether we drink coffee, what medicines we take, and whether we exercise and more!
- It has been postulated that an alteration in gut microbiota plays a seminal role in the development of obesity and type 2 diabetes.
- There are innumerable potential medical applications based on our ongoing understanding of the microbiome. Research is being conducted in renowned academic centers throughout the world, and we will likely see major therapeutic advances in many chronic disorders including autism, cancer, autoimmune diseases and even COVID-19. We may well live longer as well!

7

DIABETES AND CARDIOVASCULAR DISEASE

> *Diabetes just boggles me. I know when you get a heart pain; I've had them. I don't know what diabetes feels like. ... If someone had said to me, 'What's your number one health problem?', I would have said heart disease and then diabetes. And what doctors tell me now is that I can transpose them and say diabetes first.*
>
> —Larry King

Cardiovascular disease is a major cause of both morbidity and mortality in people with diabetes, and most people (up to 70%) with diabetes will die of cardiovascular disease.

Diabetes is such a strong contributor to cardiovascular disease that it is considered a **cardiovascular risk equivalent**. This means that it is a significant independent risk factor for cardiovascular disease. In other words, it is a risk factor just like high blood pressure (hypertension), high blood cholesterol and lipids (hyperlipidemia) and smoking; it's presence significantly increases the risk of developing heart disease.

In fact, people with type 2 diabetes who have never had a myocardial infarction (a heart attack) are at the same risk of having one as someone who has already had one. This was shown by Haffner and colleagues over 20 years ago in a landmark article published in the *New England Journal of Medicine* in 1998. Another important recent study, the Framingham heart study, also showed that the presence of diabetes *doubled* the risk for cardiovascular disease in men and *tripled* it in women. This increase in risk is also because people with diabetes are more likely to have hypertension and hyperlipidemia.

Unfortunately, diabetes also increases the likelihood of developing the complications of cardiovascular disease, including heart failure. It is also associated with fewer symptoms of coronary artery disease. This

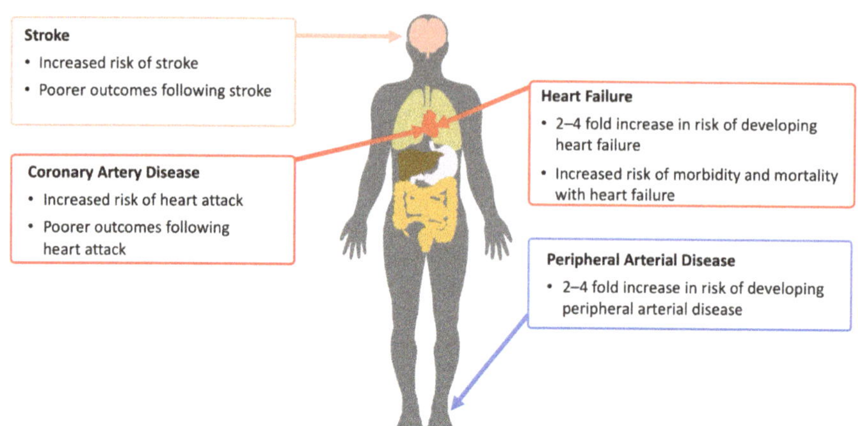

Poorly controlled diabetes causes an increase in atherosclerosis, the formation of plaques in the walls of the larger blood vessels, including arteries and blood vessels in the brain, heart and limbs. This decreases their elasticity and blood flow downstream and increases the risk of strokes and heart attacks caused by lumps of the plaque breaking off and blocking arteries of the brain and heart. Adapted from the ASCEND (Academy for Science and Continuing Education in Diabetes and Obesity) Program. http://www.ASCEND-diabetes-obesity.com.

might sound a positive thing, but it actually means that disease can progress, undetected, to a more severe state. For example, people with diabetes are often surprised to find that they have previously had a "silent heart attack" when an electrocardiogram (EKG) is done during a routine office visit.

This "silence" is thought to be related to how diabetes damages nerves, including those of the autonomic nervous system, which controls fundamental physiology such as heart rate and blood pressure. This **autonomic neuropathy** (see page 67) can also contribute to irregular heart rhythms (cardiac arrhythmias) such as atrial fibrillation, which in turn increase the risk of cardiovascular and cerebrovascular disease, such as stroke.

Cardiovascular Risk Factors

People with type 2 diabetes are more likely to have other cardiovascular risk factors, notably hypertension and dyslipidemia, as they have shared causes such as diet and lifestyle. This means all these risk factors need to be treated aggressively to prevent cardiovascular disease starting or getting worse.

The good news is that there has been a significant decline in rates of myocardial infarction in people with diabetes over the years. This is in large part due to the widespread introduction and use of powerful medications like statins for high cholesterol and antihypertensives for lowering blood pressure. The 2008 Steno 2 study compared the intensive treatment of multiple cardiovascular risk factors versus conventional treatment. In those treated aggressively, there was an astounding 50% reduction in risk for cardiovascular events (such as angina), including death from cardiovascular disease!

> In the Steno 2 study, published in the *New England Journal of Medicine* in 2008 people with type 2 diabetes were randomized to receive intensive multiple risk factor modification treatment versus conventional treatment. In those treated aggressively there was an astounding 50% reduction in risk for cardiovascular events and even death from cardiovascular disease.

The people who participated in the Steno 2 study were followed closely for up to 21 years. A continued benefit was seen in those who had been treated intensively, including a 70% reduction in risk for developing heart failure and a 69% reduction in risk of a stroke. In fact, the authors noted that intensive management of all cardiovascular risk factors prolonged life by 7.9 years! These follow-up studies were published in *Diabetologia* in 2016 and 2019.

And so, the key message is that aggressive management of all cardiovascular risk factors is an essential part of diabetes care.

Aspirin

Aspirin prevents the aggregation of platelets, a key part of the formation of blood clots, and therefore cause a "thinning" of blood. This can protect against heart attacks and stroke. However, aspirin can also increase the risk of significant bleeding in the gastrointestinal tract and brain. It is therefore currently recommended that aspirin not be used routinely to prevent a heart attack in someone who has not had one, especially in people over the age of 70. However, once someone has had a heart attack, aspirin is recommended to reduce the risk of subsequent heart attacks. This is known as "secondary prevention."

Control of Blood Glucose

We now know that tight glucose control in people with newly diagnosed diabetes has a long-term benefit including reducing the risk for cardiovascular disease, even if tight glucose control cannot be maintained indefinitely. This applies to people with both type I and type 2 diabetes and was demonstrated in the long-term follow-up of two landmark trials, the Diabetes Control and Complications Trial (DCCT), for type 1 diabetes, and the United Kingdom Prospective Diabetes Study (UKPDS), which looked at type 2 diabetes (see page 143).

At the end of the initial phase of the DCCT, there was no difference seen in cardiovascular risk or mortality between the intensive insulin treatment and conventional insulin treatment groups. However, when the participants were followed-up for an additional 10 to 15 years, those who had been in the intensive treatment group demonstrated a significant reduction in risk for cardiovascular events compared to those in the conventional treatment arm, even though there was no difference in their glucose control after the study had ended.

Similarly, in the UKPDS, those randomized to intensive treatment demonstrated long-term cardiovascular benefit despite no difference in glucose control between the intensively treated and conventionally treated groups after the trial had ended. We do not understand the mechanisms underlying this fascinating "legacy effect" (or "memory effect"). Somehow, good glucose control for some years after initial diagnosis confers a long-term benefit!

Improving Glucose Control in Long-term, High-risk Patients

What about people who have had type 2 diabetes for many years, have not had optimal control and who are at high risk for cardiovascular disease? Or those who have already developed cardiovascular disease? Does improving their glucose control improve cardiovascular outcomes?

Three major trials have addressed this:

1. ACCORD (Action to Control Cardiovascular Risk in Diabetes).
2. ADVANCE (Action in Diabetes and Vascular Disease).
3. VADT (Veterans Administration Diabetes Trial).

They all showed similar results – improving glucose control did **not** confer any cardiovascular benefit, but it **did** reduce the risk for the development or progression of kidney disease or retinopathy.

There are now two classes of drugs that have been shown to have cardiovascular benefit independent of their glucose lowering effects. They are GLP-1 receptor agonists and SGLT-2 inhibitors.

Other Strategies to Improve Cardiovascular Health

Aside from treating diabetes, hypertension, hyperlipidemia and stopping smoking, what other interventions might reduce cardiovascular disease in people with diabetes? Several observational studies from various parts of the world have shown that regular exercise (e.g., in one study it was walking for two hours per week) significantly reduces cardiovascular events and mortality.

In the Physicians Health Study, people with diabetes who consumed a moderate amount of alcohol on a regular basis had a lower risk of death from cardiovascular disease than people who did not.

Finally, stress reduction may also help prevent cardiovascular disease. In a recent paper published in the *Journal of the American Heart Association* in 2017, Levine and colleagues commented that regular meditation has been shown to produce certain neuroanatomical and neurophysiological benefits, and suggested that this may help reduce cardiovascular events but that more studies are needed to confirm the benefit.

Medications That Lower Cardiovascular Risk

In 2009, the Federal Drug Administration (FDA) mandated that any new class of drugs being developed for people with type 2 diabetes had to be evaluated for cardiovascular risk as well. Many of these studies were conducted in people who had established cardiovascular disease or were at high risk for the development cardiovascular disease.

There are now two classes of drugs that have been shown to have a cardiovascular benefit independent of their glucose-lowering effects. They are the glucagon-like peptide-1 (GLP-1) receptor agonists (see page 154) and the sodium-glucose cotransporter-2 (SGLT-2) inhibitors (see page 156). SGLT-2 inhibitors have also been shown to reduce the need for hospitalization and lower mortality in people with heart failure, and to slow the rate of progression of kidney dysfunction. This has been heralded as one of the most exciting advances in the management of diabetes in the past 25 years.

Patient Stories: Cardiovascular Complications 1

CC is a 70-year-old man who has had type 2 diabetes for 15 years. He has had no complications related to diabetes other than coronary artery disease which manifested as a heart attack five years ago. He used to smoke a pack of cigarettes a day and stopped after his heart attack. He walks four times per week for up to 30 minutes and avoids too many carbohydrates in his diet. He has lost 15 pounds [6.8 kg] since his heart attack. Six months ago, he began to experience episodes of shortness of breath, especially at night, and presented to the emergency room on four separate occasions where he required oxygen and some medications (diuretics) to relieve the symptoms. A diagnosis of congestive heart failure was made.

His diabetes medications are metformin, a sulfonylurea and basal insulin. He also takes other medications for elevated cholesterol (a statin) and high blood pressure (an angiotensin converting enzyme (ACE) inhibitor) as well as aspirin and a diuretic.

He tests his blood sugars at least three times per day – in the morning, before lunch or dinner and at bedtime, and they are usually in the 90 to 180 mg/dL range (5 to 10 mmol/L). His most recent HbA1c was 7.5%.

When one of us saw him, we discussed with him the recent data showing the benefit of SGLT-2 inhibitors in people with heart failure. He was prescribed one of these and the sulfonylurea was stopped. He also agreed to continue to try to improve his exercise routine and to adhere more stringently to his diet.

When seen three months later, he came into the office beaming and proudly announced that he had not experienced any episodes of shortness of breath, even while walking, and that he had not needed to go to the emergency room even once. He was now walking six days a week and his most recent blood glucose levels, tested before meals, ranged from 90 to 165 mg/dL (5 to 9 mmol/L). His repeat HbA1c was now 7.2%. He had also lost another 4 pounds [1.8 kg].

Take-Home Message

The take-home message from this patient's story is that this new class of medication (first approved for use in the United States by the FDA in 2013) has significant benefits beyond just lowering glucose, in that they lower the risk of hospitalization for heart failure and even the risk of death from cardiovascular disease.

Patient Stories: Cardiovascular Complications 2

DL is a 55-year-old woman who has had type 2 diabetes for 12 years, since she was 43. She had struggled with weight issues for many years, having gained 30 pounds]13.6 kg] in the last ten years. She ascribed this to worsening pain in both knees due to osteoarthritis.

She, like many others, was able to initially control her glucose levels without insulin. However, with the weight gain and ongoing duration of diabetes, she was started on insulin four years ago and subsequently required both basal and prandial insulin (rapid-acting insulin with meals). Of more concern to her was the fact that the doses of insulin had to be increased to achieve optimal glucose control.

Approximately five years ago, she presented to the emergency room with severe chest pain. An emergency cardiac catheterization was performed and revealed critical narrowing of three coronary arteries. The cardiologist deployed three stents in those arteries to improve blood flow to the heart muscle.

Since then, she has had no further episodes of chest pain and manages to swim for 30 minutes, four times a week.

She was referred by her primary care physician, who asked if there was anything we could recommend to reduce her doses of insulin.

We discussed the singular benefits of two classes of relatively new medications - GLP-1 receptor agonists and SGLT-2 inhibitors - and the impressive studies showing that these medications lowered the risk of cardiovascular events, which can be life-threatening. These pronounced benefits are seen even if there are no improvements in blood glucose levels.

She was prescribed a GLP-1 receptor agonist, which she injected once a week. At the same time, she reduced the doses of insulin. One month later she reported that she was able to maintain lower doses of insulin, that her glucose levels were "excellent" and that she had lost 4 pounds [1.8 kg]. She did experience a side effect - mild nausea, which is seen in about 10% of people who start this new medication. Fortunately, she was able to tolerate it and the nausea abated after four weeks.

One year later she continues to improve. She stopped taking rapid-acting insulin at meals eight months ago and has maintained excellent glucose control. She has had no episodes of chest pain. She has lost another 10 pounds [4.5 kg], some of which can be ascribed as a documented benefit of this class of drugs. This is remarkable, considering some drugs used to treat diabetes can lead to weight *gain*!

Take-Home Messages

- She was able to stop the insulin at meals and is taking fewer injections!
- She tolerated the medication well and the initial nausea abated over a 4-week period.
- She has lost weight, some of which can be ascribed to the medication.
- She is taking a medication that is known to decrease the frequency of major cardiovascular events, such as heart attack and even cardiovascular death.

Strategies To Reduce Cardiovascular Risk

The ten core strategies to reduce cardiovascular risk are:

1. Control of high blood pressure.
2. Control of elevated cholesterol.
3. Control of high blood glucose.
4. Cessation of smoking.
5. Regular exercise.
6. Stress reduction.
7. Losing excess weight.
8. Healthy dietary habits.
9. Judicious use of certain glucose lowering medications that also reduce cardiovascular mortality.
10. Aspirin for secondary prevention of heart attacks.

Long-Term Benefits of Intensive Multifactorial Intervention

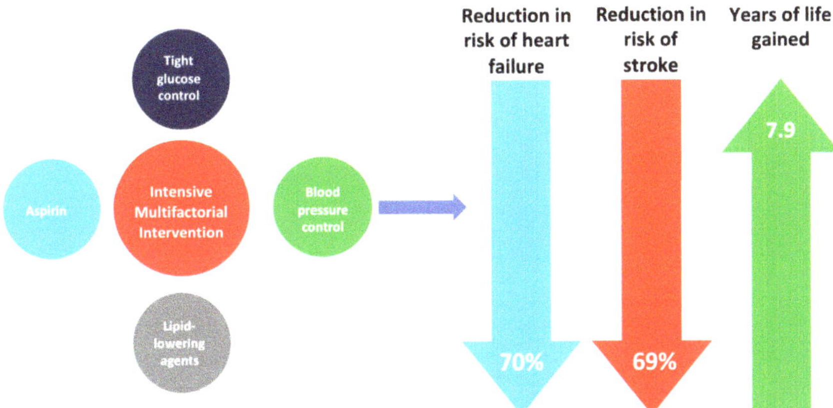

Intensive multifactorial intervention continues to have long-term benefits after more than 20 years. Adapted from the ASCEND (Academy for Science and Continuing Education in Diabetes and Obesity) Program. http://www.ASCEND-diabetes-obesity.com.

Key Points

- Good glucose control matters, regardless of whether you are newly diagnosed or if you have had diabetes for many years.
- Aggressive management – for the most part pharmacological – of all cardiovascular risk factors including hypertension, hyperlipidemia and smoking cessation is of paramount importance if you want to reduce your risk for cardiovascular disease.
- There are new medications to treat diabetes – GLP-1 receptor agonists and SGLT-2 inhibitors – that also confer significant cardiovascular benefit. This has been a "game changer" in clinical practice. If you have cardiovascular disease, you should be taking at least one of these to further lower cardiovascular risk.
- Regular exercise and moderate alcohol intake have cardiovascular benefit.
- Stress reduction is beneficial – regular meditation has many health benefits, one of which may be reduction in cardiovascular risk.
- Finally, low-dose aspirin is still recommended for people with established cardiovascular disease, but not necessarily for the prevention of cardiovascular disease, since aspirin use has been linked to a slight but significant increased risk for bleeding, particularly in people over 70.

8

COMPLICATIONS OF DIABETES: RETINOPATHY

The only thing worse than being blind is having sight but no vision.

—Helen Keller

We mentioned previously that diabetes can affect both the small and large blood vessels, causing microvascular and macrovascular disease, respectively. The organs of the body most susceptible to microvascular disease are the eye, peripheral nerves (i.e., those of the extremities) and the kidneys, leading to diabetic retinopathy (this chapter), diabetic neuropathy and foot problems (chapter 9, page 65) and diabetic nephropathy (chapter 10, page 71), respectively. There is nothing "micro" about the health effects of diabetic microvascular disease; diabetes is the commonest cause of blindness, end-stage renal disease and non-traumatic lower limb amputations in the western world.

Macrovascular disease primarily affects the large vessels of the heart, brain, legs, and feet. Having diabetes *doubles your risk for a heart attack and almost doubles it for stroke.*

How Diabetes Causes Retinal Disease

Diabetes affects the small blood vessels in the retina, the complex, delicate and light-sensitive lining at the back of the eye essential for vision. Damage to these blood vessels reduces oxygen supply to the retina. As a result, some vessels swell and leak fluid, other areas of the retina become completely starved of oxygen, and new blood vessels begin to grow in an attempt to compensate. The risk for developing retinopathy increases with the duration of diabetes. It is estimated that up to 90% of people with type 1 diabetes will develop retinopathy. Fortunately, in most instances, it is mild and asymptomatic.

Types of Diabetic Retinopathy

There are two main forms of retinopathy - **non-proliferative** and **proliferative**. "Proliferative" is more serious but much less common, and describes the presence of new blood vessels, which are delicate and prone to leaking blood. These "hemorrhages" lead to impaired vision and the need for specific treatments.

In the early stages of retinopathy, there are no symptoms at all. It is only in the late, proliferative stages that there may be symptoms. These include low vision or seeing floating spots or streaks. Severe retinopathy can lead to blindness if not treated.

In people with type 1 diabetes, the risk of developing retinopathy begins more than five years after a diagnosis of diabetes. However, in people with type 2 diabetes, retinopathy may be present at the time of diagnosis. This is because many people with type 2 diabetes may have had diabetes for many years before being diagnosed.

> The late Judah Folkman, a brilliant scientist who worked at Boston Children's Hospital and Harvard Medical School, spawned an entirely new medical field in the study of **angiogenesis**. Angiogenesis is the formation of new blood vessels, as seen in proliferative retinopathy, and it is also important in cancer biology, as it is a key trait of malignant tumors to recruit and grow new blood vessels to fuel their growth and spread.

How to Reduce Your Risk

The risk for the development or progression of diabetic retinopathy is significantly lower in people who can maintain good glucose control after diagnosis. Two seminal studies shed light on this.

The first was the landmark Diabetes Control and Complications Trial (DCCT) which was undertaken in people with type 1 diabetes, and which was published in the *New England Journal of Medicine* in 1993. The second study which changed the clinical care of people with type 2 diabetes was the United Kingdom Prospective Diabetes Study (UKPDS), published in the *Lancet* in 1998.

Long-term data showed that within a year of completion of these studies the people in both treatment groups (intensive vs standard care) had identical HbA1c levels. Interestingly, long-term follow-up showed that those who were originally in the intensive treatment group continued to show less risk for the onset or progression of retinopathy even though their glucose control was no different from the control group.

The Laser Age

Today there is very effective treatment for severe retinopathy. Laser photocoagulation therapy was first developed in the 1960s and led to a remarkable reduction in blindness from retinopathy. It involves using a laser to destroy or seal the unwanted, leaky new vessels seen in proliferative retinopathy.

Everyone is familiar with the word, but many may not be aware that "laser" is an acronym: *Light Amplification by Stimulated Emission of Radiation*. The concepts of laser were first developed by Albert Einstein in 1917.

In the late 1940s researchers described retinal photocoagulation with a form of laser but it was difficult to use in clinical practice. A little bit more than a decade later, in 1960, American physicist Theodore Maiman created the first working laser with a ruby crystal medium. This heralded the dawn for laser treatments in ophthalmic conditions.

The first laser to be used to treat early proliferative diabetic retinopathy was ruby laser photocoagulation and was performed by William Beetham and his son-in-law Lloyd M. Aiello at the Joslin Clinic in 1969. Two important large, multicenter, randomized clinical trials were subsequently conducted and led to the development of guidelines for laser treatment of proliferative retinopathy. In one of these studies (the Diabetic Retinopathy Study) panretinal laser photocoagulation reduced the risk of severe visual loss by more than 50% at the 5-year follow up.

VEGF Inhibitors

More recently, new medications called vascular endothelial growth factor (VEGF) inhibitors have become available. They are injected into the back of the eye and inhibit the growth of new blood vessels. In fact, they have been shown to be even more effective than laser treatment.

In recent years VEGF inhibitors have been found to be very effective in people with prolifcrative retinopathy and swelling (edema) in the central and visually important part of the retina called the macula. They are now the first line standard treatment in many parts of the world.

Thanks to these two innovative treatments, the risk of blindness from retinopathy is currently less than 4%. In fact, diabetes is now no longer the leading cause of blindness in England and Wales because of aggressive screening and treatment programs. This was eloquently reviewed by Jampol and colleagues in a 2020 review article in the *New England Journal of Medicine.*

Other Eye Problems in Diabetes

People with diabetes may also develop other eye problems which may lead to significant visual impairment. These include cataract, glaucoma and age-related macular degeneration.

Reducing Your Risk for Diabetic Retinopathy

Maintaining good glucose control is the single most important factor. Good glucose control reduces the risk for the development or progression of complications like retinopathy. It is also important to make sure that your blood pressure and cholesterol levels are also well-controlled, since high blood pressure and elevated cholesterol levels also increase the risk of eye complications. Most importantly, you should have regular, annual dilated eye examinations with an experienced ophthalmologist or optometrist.

People with type 2 diabetes should have an eye exam at the time of diagnosis and annually thereafter; screening for retinopathy for people with type 1 diabetes should start five years after diagnosis. In addition to the dilated eye exam, your doctor should also check your intraocular pressure (to assess for glaucoma) and evaluate you for cataracts.

Future Studies

What does the future portend? There have been major advances in the development of imaging techniques to screen for retinopathy. Patients also have greater access to these modalities; use of mobile vans in communities facilitate this. Additionally, artificial intelligence (AI) can be applied to diagnose and identify patients who need referral for retinal examination and potentially sight-saving therapy.

Patient Stories: Unexpected Retinopathy

Ms. R is a 62-year-old woman with newly diagnosed type 2 diabetes. This was diagnosed during a routine annual checkup. As part of her comprehensive evaluation, she was referred to an ophthalmologist for a dilated eye examination to assess if she had any damage to her retina, though she had no visual complaints.

To her surprise the ophthalmologist found moderately severe retinopathy which, if left untreated, could lead to significant loss of vision. The medical diagnosis was "severe non proliferative retinopathy with macular edema of both eyes."

She was treated with a course of intraocular injections of a VEGF inhibitor. These medications have been shown to significantly prevent and even reverse visual loss in people with diabetic retinopathy.

At a six-month follow-up she was re-evaluated and was overjoyed to hear that the medications had worked well, and that the macular edema had resolved completely.

Take-Home Message

Diabetic retinopathy is often asymptomatic and yet can lead to significant visual loss. Hence the importance of ophthalmic evaluation at the time of diagnosis and annually thereafter.

Key Points

- The risk for the development or progression of diabetic retinopathy is significantly lower in people who can maintain good glucose control after diagnosis.
- With the use of laser photocoagulation and VEGF inhibitors, the risk of blindness from retinopathy is currently less than 4%.
- Artificial intelligence (AI) can be applied to diagnose and identify patients who need referral for retinal examination and potentially sight saving therapy.

9

COMPLICATIONS OF DIABETES: NEUROPATHY AND THE DIABETIC FOOT

I had the blues because I had no shoes until upon the street, I met a man who had no feet.

—Denis W. Waitley

Along with microvascular disease affecting the retina and the kidney, another microvascular complication of diabetes is nerve damage, or neuropathy. There are various types that can affect people with diabetes, but the commonest is **peripheral neuropathy** (also called polyneuropathy) that affects the nerves that supply sensation to the feet. Neuropathy occurs in people with both type 1 and type 2 diabetes, and the prevalence varies according to the duration of diabetes and the degree of hyperglycemia. After 25 years of diabetes, approximately 50% of people will have some manifestations of neuropathy, which can range from very mild to severe.

How Diabetes Causes Neuropathy

Over time high blood glucose levels weaken the walls of small blood vessels, known as capillaries, by a mixture of mechanisms including oxidative stress and glucose disrupting proteins in the capillary walls. These vessels supply oxygen and other nutrients to the nerves, and as they fail, so do the nerves they supply. The most vulnerable nerves are those furthest from the heart, where blood supply is scarcer, and so the nerves of the feet are usually affected first, leading to peripheral neuropathy of the feet.

Signs and Symptoms

The commonest signs of neuropathy include diminished sensation, numbness, or tingling in the feet. Some people develop pain in the feet, which is often worse at night, and other people may complain of an altered sensation in their feet when walking, often described as if they are walking on coals. Painful neuropathy associated with diabetes may significantly impact on quality of life and is unfortunately an extremely challenging condition to treat and manage effectively.

If the neuropathy worsens these abnormal symptoms may progress up the legs and even sometimes into the hands.

Complications

When sensation is diminished in the foot, there is increased risk for damage to the skin, and even to the muscles, ligaments and bones of the feet. For example, if somebody with neuropathy cuts their foot and does not sense there is a cut, the cut can become infected, and the infection can spread and become serious if not treated.

People with neuropathy are at increased risk for the development of ulcers, which are more likely to occur on sites of higher pressure on the feet. These too can become infected, and these infections can even spread to the bones of the feet, a very serious condition called **osteomyelitis**. If this occurs, aggressive treatment with antibiotics is required, and if the infection cannot be controlled, amputation of toes or part of the foot may be necessary. Approximately 20% of people with diabetes who develop a foot ulcer are likely to require some form of amputation.

We also mentioned that the larger blood vessels can be affected by diabetes, and the larger blood vessels that supply oxygen to the legs and feet are no exception. This peripheral vascular disease, due to atherosclerosis in the large arteries of the leg, limits blood flow downstream. Combined with the decreased sensation due to neuropathy, this increases the risk of infection and gangrene, which may also lead to amputation.

Ultimately, through damage to the bones, tendons and ligaments of the foot, neuropathy can lead to alteration in the shape of the foot, known as **Charcot foot**, and further risk for ulcer development and infection.

The Importance of Foot Care

Care of your feet is particularly important if you have diabetes. It is important to wear shoes that are well fitting, avoid walking anywhere barefoot (particularly outdoors) and to do whatever possible to reduce the risk for of any sores or cuts. Regular examination by a podiatrist is also important (see the checklist on page 219).

Once again, as with all complications of diabetes, it is good glucose control that reduces the risk for the development or progression of neuropathy.

Other Types of Diabetic Neuropathy

There are other, less common forms of neuropathy that can affect people with diabetes. They may include damage to the autonomic nervous system; the part of the nervous system responsible that controls essential functions that are not consciously directed, such as breathing, the heartbeat, and digestive processes.

Autonomic neuropathy in someone with diabetes can result in an increased risk for cardiac arrhythmias, and symptoms of dizziness when standing, called orthostatic hypotension. It can also affect nerves related to the gastrointestinal system, leading to constipation or diarrhea. The diarrhea is often worse at night.

Neuropathy can also affect larger nerves of the body, and even some individual nerves that supply large or small muscles, including muscles of the eye. Interestingly, some of these forms of neuropathy affecting only a single nerve (**mononeuropathy**) tend to resolve spontaneously over time.

Nerve conduction studies are tests that can be done to confirm neuropathy in the outpatient setting, but the diagnosis is most often made based on clinical symptoms and signs.

Treatment

Once again, the best treatment is prevention, achieved by maintaining good blood glucose control.

If painful neuropathy occurs, there are medications that can be taken to relieve the pain. In addition, a topical medication called capsaicin was approved by the FDA in July 2020 for the treatment of painful neuropathy.

If you have neuropathy and decreased sensation in your feet, it is important to both avoid anything that can lead to damage to the foot and to have your feet checked regularly by your doctor or a podiatrist.

If you have neuropathy and decreased sensation in your feet, it is important to both avoid anything that can lead to damage to the foot and to have your feet checked regularly by your doctor or a podiatrist.

Other Causes of Neuropathy

It is also important to remember that there are other causes of peripheral neuropathy that can affect people with diabetes. These include hereditary forms, vitamin B 12 deficiency, alcohol, certain chemotherapeutic drugs, and some infections. Although diabetes is the most common cause of neuropathy in someone with diabetes, be sure that your physician rules out other causes of neuropathy before diagnosing it as due to diabetes.

How to Prevent Nerve Damage in Diabetes

- Optimal control of blood glucose levels.
- Smoking cessation.
- Optimal control of blood pressure.
- Optimal control of blood lipids (cholesterol and triglycerides).
- Optimal weight.

Patient Stories: Not All Neuropathy is Diabetic....

PN is a 62-year-old Asian American woman who has had type 2 diabetes for three years. Her medical history is only remarkable for having had gastroesophageal reflux disease (GERD; heartburn) for the last ten years. Her blood glucose has been well-controlled on metformin and the heartburn by a proton pump inhibitor which she takes daily.

She came to see one of us complaining that she was experiencing some numbness and tingling in her feet. She said, "I always feel as if I am walking on pebbles and this tingling often keeps me up at night." She wondered if this was related to her diabetes because she has a friend with type 2 diabetes who complained of similar symptoms.

A clinical diagnosis of peripheral neuropathy was made. It was noted that her diabetes was well controlled – her recent HbA1c was 6.5% and it had not exceeded 6.8% in the last two years. Considering this, we discussed other potential causes of peripheral neuropathy, and it occurred to us that both medications she was taking (metformin and the proton pump inhibitor) can rarely lead to vitamin B12 deficiency, a cause of peripheral neuropathy independent of diabetes.

A blood test was drawn to measure the vitamin B12 level. The result confirmed marked deficiency. She was started on treatment with vitamin B12 and when seen three months later, she commented that the annoying symptoms of numbness and tingling had totally resolved!

Take-Home Messages

- Peripheral neuropathy is a common condition with different causes, some of which are completely reversible.
- Just because someone has diabetes and now develops classical peripheral neuropathy does not mean that it is due to the diabetes.
- There are commonly used medications such as metformin, proton pump inhibitors, colchicine (a medication often used to treat gout) and alcohol which can also cause B12 deficiency.

Key Points

- Approximately 20% of people with diabetes who develop a foot ulcer are likely to require some form of amputation.
- It is important to remember that there are other, non-diabetic causes of peripheral neuropathy that can affect people with diabetes. These include hereditary forms, vitamin B 12 deficiency, alcohol, certain chemotherapeutic drugs, and some infections.
- For those with peripheral neuropathy, it is important to wear shoes that are well-fitting, avoid walking barefoot anywhere (particularly outdoors) and to do whatever is possible to avoid getting sores or cuts on their feet.

10

COMPLICATIONS OF DIABETES: NEPHROPATHY

For diabetes in particular, we know there's a relationship between lack of glucose regulation and complications like blindness and kidney failure. So, if you were diabetic and you knew that you could get your glucose in a tight, normal range just by adjusting your lifestyle, wouldn't that be great....?

—Eric Topol, MD

Diabetes is the leading cause of chronic kidney disease and end-stage kidney disease (ESKD) in the United States and worldwide. Approximately one third of people with diabetes will develop kidney disease, but not all of those who develop kidney disease progress to ESKD. People with ESKD often need long-term dialysis or renal transplantation.

Although both are lifesaving treatments, dialysis is intensely demanding and significantly and negatively alters the quality of a patient's life. Kidney transplantation, on the other hand, results in a significant improvement in the quality of life. However, the average waiting time for a person to receive a kidney transplant is long. In the U.S, for example, it is five years after a diagnosis of ESKD.

How Diabetes Causes Nephropathy

In poorly controlled diabetes, damage occurs over time to the relatively delicate clusters of blood vessels in the kidneys that filter waste products from the blood to produce urine. As it worsens, it can lead to increased blood pressure and, eventually, kidney failure.

Diagnosis

The diagnosis of diabetic kidney disease is usually made on clinical grounds, although occasionally a kidney biopsy is done to look for characteristic changes under the microscope.

In the early 1980's it was noticed that the urine of some patients with diabetes contained albumin, a small blood protein. This leakage of albumin – which as a valuable protein is not meant to be lost in urine! – represents damage to the sensitive filtering membrane of the kidney, between the blood and the urine, allowing it to "leak" through.

It was often present in small amounts in those with diabetes, and hence the term microalbuminuria was adopted. It is now referred to as moderately increased albuminuria because there was confusion that the term "microalbuminuria" implied a different kind of albumin. It is now known that the presence of albumin in the urine of someone with diabetes predicts a higher future risk of both kidney disease and cardiovascular disease in the patient.

If there is a lot of albumin in the urine, it is referred to as severely increased albuminuria and it forecasts an even more serious prognosis.

In addition to testing the urine for the presence of albumin or protein, estimation of kidney function is routinely and reliably done by clinicians. This is a routine laboratory test done on a blood sample.

Recent studies have shed light on the natural history of albuminuria in people with diabetes. Remarkably, in some people the leakage of

The Progression of Chronic Kidney Disease in Diabetes

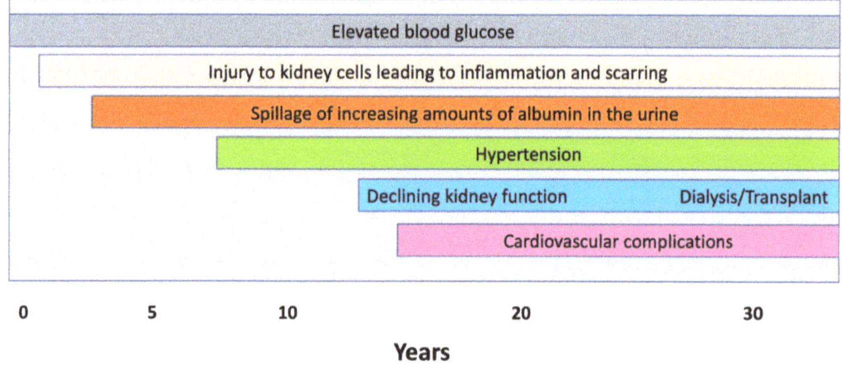

moderate or large amounts of the protein albumin into the urine may *regress*. This is associated with a more favorable prognosis than might have been originally assumed.

Reducing Your Risk

The risk for progression to ESKD is variable and depends on several factors. These include the type of diabetes (type 1 or 2), other coexisting medical conditions, notably high blood pressure, genetic factors (for example, African Americans are at greater risk) and the use and efficacy of dietary and pharmaceutical interventions. The use of certain antihypertensives (angiotensin-converting enzyme (ACE) inhibitors and angiotensin receptor blockers) reduces the rate of progression of kidney disease and may even reverse albuminuria in its early stages. Good blood glucose control also reduces the risk of progression.

The recently introduced sodium-glucose cotransporter-2 (SGLT-2) inhibitors, used to lower blood glucose in treatment of type 2 diabetes (see page 156), have also been shown to slow the rate of progression of kidney disease.

In addition, we encourage our patients to quit smoking if they are doing so, to curtail alcohol intake and to exercise regularly. Interestingly, coffee drinkers have been shown to have less progression of their chronic kidney disease compared to non-coffee drinkers!

Cardiovascular complications are more frequent in patients with albuminuria. It is critical for patients with diabetes and kidney disease to be seen by their primary care clinician, nephrologist (kidney specialist) and nutritionist on an ongoing basis.

For many years it was thought that elevated blood levels of uric acid were associated with an increased risk for progression of diabetic kidney disease. Medications can be used to lower uric acid levels. However, a 2020 study published in the *New England Journal of Medicine* looked at the effect of a uric acid lowering medication called allopurinol on the progression of kidney disease in people with diabetes. They found that lowering uric acid levels did not alter the progression. The study was conducted in older people with quite advanced renal disease, and whether lowering uric acid would be beneficial in younger individuals with less advanced kidney disease remains to be determined.

Patient Stories: Long-standing Type 2 Diabetes and Kidney Problems

STK is a 66-year-old African American man who recently retired after serving 40 years in the coastguard. He has had type 2 diabetes for 20 years and was initially treated with diet and exercise but then required medications, including metformin and a sulfonylurea. Over the passage of time, glucose control worsened, and he was advised to start insulin. He was initially reluctant to do so, but subsequently agreed, following a thorough review of all his test results and the treatment options for him.

Five years ago, he was diagnosed with mild non-proliferative retinopathy at his annual dilated eye examination. No treatment for this was required. At the same time, it was also noted that he had albuminuria and his blood pressure was elevated. His kidney function was mildly impaired. He was advised to adhere to his treatment regimen, with an aim of good control of both blood sugar and blood pressure to slow the rate of progression of his kidney disease. He was then seen by a nephrologist who ruled out non-diabetic causes of kidney dysfunction, and who reinforced the need for good glucose and blood pressure control. The nephrologist also tested vitamin D and parathyroid hormone levels to make sure these were normal, to rule out a condition called secondary hyperparathyroidism. He was found to be vitamin D deficient and was started on vitamin D supplementation.

Since then, he has maintained meticulous glucose and blood pressure control. His vitamin D and parathyroid levels are normal. There has been only a slight deterioration in his kidney function and the amount of albumin in the urine has been stable and not increased. He continues to see the nephrologist regularly. Recently he was started on a SGLT-2 inhibitor since these medications have been shown to slow the rate of progression of kidney disease in people with diabetes.

Take-Home Messages

- The risk for the development of microvascular complications of diabetes increases with time, especially if glucose control is not optimal.
- It is never too late to work on improving glucose control! Even if you have had diabetes for many years, improving glucose control can slow the rate of progression of kidney disease.

- Treatment of other factors that can lead to progression of kidney disease is very important – these include high blood pressure and ensuring normal vitamin D and parathyroid levels.
- Other specialists, in this case nephrologists, play a very important role in managing people with diabetic nephropathy and should have ongoing consultation in patients with this disease.

Patient Stories: The Amazing Kidney Donation Chain

Rick Ruzzamenti (RR) was always impulsive. He converted to Buddhism in a flash and married a Vietnamese woman whom he had only known for a short time.

He used to regularly go to a yoga studio. He had not seen the desk clerk for a while and when she returned, he asked her if everything was OK? She replied that she had donated a kidney to an ailing friend whom she had recently bumped into at a department store.

The story so captivated RR, who was 44 at the time, that although he had never even donated blood, he called the Riverside Community Hospital in California and said, "I want to donate a kidney"!

He was evaluated at the hospital and subsequently told that he was not a suitable match for any of the patients on their waiting list. Again, impulsively he said, "If I am not suitable for any of your patients, what about patients at other nearby hospitals?"

This started an amazing chain reaction. Over a 4-month period in 17 hospitals in 11 US states, something phenomenal happened. Thirty healthy donors donated a kidney to thirty recipients. Sixty people thereby inextricably linked.

This story is told in a fascinating article in the *New York Times* of February 18th, 2012. It has every donor and each recipient's photograph, apart from one person who chose not to have their picture in the article. Children donated for parents, husbands for wives, sisters for brothers.

This has been called the kidney transplant chain. RR started this – it was not initiated by the transplant surgeons, nephrologists, or social workers. What started this domino effect of 60 operations was the willingness of a Good Samaritan (RR) to give the initial kidney, expecting nothing in return. The momentum was swift and enormously impressive. It was predicated by both selflessness and self-interest among donors who gave a kidney to a stranger after discovering that were not suitable donors for a loved one because test results showed that they were incompatible, and it could lead to the transplanted kidney being rejected. So, they instead donated their kidneys to strangers and their loved ones, in turn, were offered compatible kidneys from other strangers as part of this exchange.

Each of the donor-patient stories are compelling, but we want to share one in particular. A patient in Illinois had diabetes-related kidney disease diagnosed in his mid 40s. He received dialysis but did not tolerate it well. His family members were either unsuitable donors or unwilling to give him a kidney. His doctors told him that the waiting list was long, and it might well take five years before he would receive a kidney transplant. He said, "It was like being sentenced to prison – like I had done something wrong in my life and this was the outcome."

Soon afterwards, he received a kidney transplant at Loyola University Medical Center. He did not get it from RR, but as the *New York Times* article states eloquently, "the two men will forever share a connection. They were the first and last people in this longest chain of kidney transplants ever constructed."

Take-Home Message

Our patients continue to inspire us!

Key Points

- To reduce the risk of diabetic nephropathy, we encourage our patients to quit smoking if they are doing so, to curtail alcohol intake and to exercise regularly. Of interest, coffee drinkers have been noted to have less progression of their chronic kidney disease as compared to non-coffee drinkers.
- Improving glucose control, even in people who have had type 2 diabetes for many years, slows the rate of progression of nephropathy.
- SGLT-2 inhibitors reduce the rate of progression of chronic kidney disease in people with diabetes.
- Cardiovascular complications are more frequent in patients with albuminuria. It is critical for patients with diabetes and kidney disease to be seen by their primary care clinician, nephrologist (kidney specialist) and nutritionist on an ongoing basis.

11

DIABETES AND LIVER DISEASE

There, inside, you filter and apportion,
you separate and divide,
you multiply and lubricate,
you raise and gather
the threads and the grams of life,
the final distillate, the intimate essences.

—"Ode to the Liver"
(excerpt) Pablo Neruda,
Nobel Laureate

Chronic liver disease and diabetes both afflict millions of people worldwide. Diabetes is associated with many liver disorders. The four main chronic liver diseases that can affect people with diabetes are alcohol-related liver disease, chronic hepatitis C, hemochromatosis and non-alcoholic fatty-liver disease. In some cases, diabetes increases the risk of liver disease, and in others, diabetes and liver disease co-occur due to shared underlying mechanisms, such as obesity and metabolic syndrome.

Alcohol-Related Liver Disease

Heavy and prolonged consumption of alcohol can lead to **cirrhosis**, severe damage of the liver leading to distortion of the liver architecture. This is the major cause of morbidity and mortality from alcohol abuse, and greatly increases the risk of **hepatocellular carcinoma** (primary liver cancer).

> The strongest biological determinant of alcoholism is having a biological parent who was an alcoholic. The evidence for this came from studies in Denmark where they have a national adoption registry that was used to analyze the association.

Chronic high alcohol intake can also lead to **chronic pancreatitis** (inflammation and damage of the pancreas) and can also adversely affect the brain and the heart, leading to a form of heart failure called

alcoholic cardiomyopathy.

The pancreas is a gland nestled behind the stomach that, as well as secreting insulin (see page 132), secretes pancreatic enzymes via a duct into the small intestine that help us digest food. Patients with chronic pancreatitis therefore often have diarrhea and an inability to digest fats, in addition to their diabetes.

Chronic Viral Hepatitis

Chronic Hepatitis C

Chronic hepatitis C virus infection afflicts an estimated 170 million individuals worldwide, while chronic hepatitis B affects 400 million: a total of over half a billion people! Both can lead to cirrhosis, primary cancer of the liver and liver failure.

In a study in 2000, Mehta and colleagues examined the prevalence of type 2 diabetes in patients with chronic hepatitis C in the United States. They reported that individuals with chronic hepatitis C who were over 40 were three times more likely to have type 2 diabetes compared with those without the infection. It has been hypothesized that the virus causes insulin resistance. Indeed, in an animal study, mice injected with the core protein of the hepatitis C virus have been shown to develop insulin resistance.

Of note, in a patient with type 2 diabetes, curing them of chronic hepatitis C often leads to an improvement in their HbA1c, and in some cases, to a complete remission of their diabetes.

Chronic Hepatitis B

What about chronic hepatitis B? An association between chronic hepatitis B infection and type 2 diabetes has been noted in some studies, but not in other well-designed studies, and therefore remains unproven.

The highest prevalence rates of chronic hepatitis B are in China, Mongolia, Vietnam, and the Philippines. Fortunately, there is a very effective vaccine. Childhood vaccination programs in Taiwan over a two-decade period led to a marked reduction in the prevalence of hepatitis B and a 75% reduction in childhood primary liver cancer mortality! This truly makes the hepatitis B vaccine the first "anti-cancer vaccine."

Patient Stories: Chronic Hepatitis C and Type 2 Diabetes

A 45-year-old white man (FH) was referred to Sanjiv for management of newly diagnosed hepatitis C infection. He was well, with no major medical problems, and was not taking any medications. He did not smoke and drank one to two whiskeys on Friday and Saturday evenings.

When he was seen in the hepatology clinic, it was discovered that he had used intravenous drugs for a 6-to-8-month period in his mid-twenties. He had shared needles with other people. Fifty percent of individuals who start using illicit intravenous drugs and sharing needles acquire acute hepatitis C within the first six months, and an astounding 75% acquire it by the end of a year. And 70% of those who acquire acute hepatitis C infection go on to become chronically infected. Thirty percent recover spontaneously.

He was fraught with remorse that he had done this decades ago and that his future was uncertain. He was now an upstanding citizen, a consultant, and married with two children. His family was tested and found to be negative. Subsequent further investigations were done, including a liver biopsy to assess the degree of liver damage. He was found to be negative for hepatitis A and B virus antibodies and received appropriate vaccinations. He stopped drinking alcohol.

The initial liver biopsy showed very mild damage, but a subsequent one done two and a half years later showed progression. We discussed treatment options and mentioned that the first treatment approved had only a 6% cure rate, but at the time he was seen, it had improved to 30%. The term "cure" is usually an overstatement for a chronic viral infection. However, hepatitis C is the only one (in humans) where it is justified. Those who have been successfully treated have no trace of the virus in their blood or liver tissue, even two decades later!

When this was mentioned to him and he was advised that more advances would occur in the next few years, he said, "I want to start the treatment now. You mentioned a 30% cure rate – for me it means 300 out of 1000 people will be cured. I am determined to be one of them!"

All the potential side effects were explained, and he was given a printed sheet listing them. He read them and said "I have one more question. Will the treatment worsen my diabetes?"

Sanjiv's response was, "There does appear to be a link. Actually, getting rid of the hepatitis C virus can sometimes lead to a marked improvement, and sometimes it can even cure the diabetes. I have had a few patients where this has happened, and in speaking to my hepatolgist (liver specialist) colleagues around the country, they have also seen this in one or two patients of theirs."

He was then treated with a 12-month regimen of Pegylated Interferon-alpha (PEG-IFN-α) and Ribavirin, the standard treatment for hepatitis C infection. Thankfully, he was cured and, six months after treatment, a hepatitis C test came back negative. He was quite emotional and gave me a hug. I met his primary care clinician four months later at a medical conference and she said, "I want to share something interesting with you. Our mutual patient now has no diabetes! He didn't lose weight or even change his diet. "Do you think this had something to do with curing his chronic hepatitis C infection?"

Currently, we have an astounding cure rate for chronic hepatitis C virus infection of 90 to 95%, even in people who also have cirrhosis or HIV infection.

Take-Home Messages

- People with type 2 diabetes should be tested for chronic hepatitis C infection.
- Since type 2 diabetes afflicts more than 450 million people worldwide and chronic hepatitis C infection is present in 170 million people in the world, many people with type 2 diabetes will also have chronic hepatitis C virus infection.
- Treatment for chronic hepatitis C virus infection has evolved over the last few decades such that the cure rate has dramatically increased from 6% to more than 90%!
- Cure of chronic hepatitis C virus infection will lead to improvement in control of type 2 diabetes or even remission/cure.

Hemochromatosis

Hemochromatosis is an inherited condition in which the gut avidly absorbs iron present in food. It is one of the most common genetic disorders in humans, with an estimated prevalence of 1 in 225 individuals of Northern European descent. It is less common in people of Black, Hispanic and Asian ancestry.

The excess iron accumulates in the liver, pancreas, heart and skin. It can lead to diabetes, cirrhosis and primary cancer of the liver, cardiomyopathy (a form of heart failure) and a bronze discoloration of the skin. Indeed, in earlier times hemochromatosis was often referred to as "bronze diabetes."

The key to management is early diagnosis and treatment before the development of diabetes and cirrhosis. Treatment with weekly phlebotomy (bloodletting) and then maintenance phlebotomy (once every three to six months) is lifesaving. Patients with hemochromatosis who do not have diabetes, do not have cirrhosis and who can have the excess iron removed by weekly phlebotomy in 18 months or less have the same survival as individuals of the same gender and age who do not have hemochromatosis. This observation was published in a study in *Gastroenterology* by Niederau and colleagues.

Unfortunately, once cirrhosis is present, removal of the excess iron does not lower the inordinate high mortality from primary liver cancer, which is as high as 30%.

Patient Stories: Hemochromatosis

GK is a 38-year-old man of Irish Celtic ancestry who was referred by his primary care physician to one of us with the tentative diagnosis of genetic hemochromatosis. He sees his primary care physician on an annual basis for routine checkups and relayed to her that his one favorite uncle, 67 years of age, was recently admitted to a hospital in Brisbane, Australia, with abdominal swelling and mild confusion. He had emigrated to Australia 20 years ago.

At that hospital admission, GK's uncle was diagnosed with cirrhosis due to hemochromatosis. He was also noted to have diabetes. He was started on treatment and told that he should contact his family members and urge them to be screened for this genetic disorder.

GK's primary care clinician had drawn tests that addressed iron overload as well as liver and kidney function tests. He was noted to have a very high iron saturation in the blood and an elevated ferritin, a marker of iron storage. His liver and kidney function tests were normal.

At our appointment, there were no clinical signs of advanced liver disease present on examination. He drank alcohol, mostly one or two cans of beer, two to three times per week. He did not take any medications, notably no vitamins containing iron. We performed a blood test to see if he had the genetic mutation for hemochromatosis. It was positive!

Since we had documented signs of hemochromatosis (the high iron saturation elevated ferritin), and he had the genetic mutation, the diagnosis of hemochromatosis was established with certainty.

He was started on a 1-unit phlebotomy regimen on a weekly basis. Removal of the blood leads to the excess iron present in the liver, pancreas, and heart to be mobilized from these organs in order to produce new red blood cells. Although "blood-letting" sounds like a medieval treatment, it is the well-proven method of treating this condition.

He had 26 units removed over a seven-month period, skipping the weeks of Thanksgiving and Christmas. He was no longer iron-overloaded and is now undergoing a 1-unit phlebotomy every four months to prevent reaccumulation of iron.

Luckily, given his age (less than 40 years), normal liver size and normal liver function tests, and his ferritin of 804 (which is elevated but less than 1000), with the excess iron safely removed, he is not going to have cirrhosis of the liver or diabetes. In fact, his life expectancy is similar to anyone of his gender and age who does not have hemochromatosis!

He was estranged with a younger sister with whom he had not spoken to for close to a decade. He reached out to her and apologized for anything he might have done to have created that situation. He told her about the diagnosis of hemochromatosis in both their uncle and himself, and urged her to get tested. She was tested and also found to have hemochromatosis and underwent phlebotomy. In her case, she was adequately "de-ironed" after only 17 units of blood had been removed. This is likely because women lose blood (and hence iron) during menstruation and iron is utilized during pregnancy. She had 3 healthy children.

Unfortunately, the Red Cross does not accept blood from people with hemochromatosis for transfusion purposes. Our patient was very unhappy about this and discovered a hospital out of state which used the blood taken at the time of phlebotomy from people with hemochromatosis for transfusion purposes. This is truly iron rich blood! He traveled for an hour and a half every Thursday afternoon for his treatment saying, " I don't want this blood to go to waste!"

This refusal by many blood centers to accept blood from people with hemochromatosis is not scientifically founded. In a seminal 2018 article by Dr. Adam C. Winters and colleagues in *Hepatology*, the authors point out that "blood from hemochromatosis patients is safe and should be allowed into the donor pool." They conclude that there is no convincing evidence to exclude this population from serving as blood donors. They also inform us about the differing policy among different countries, for example, the blood from people with hemochromatosis is used in Ireland and France, but not in Austria, Hungary, Italy and Spain. A colleague of ours once did a calculation and concluded that, in the US, if all this blood taken from people with hemochromatosis was utilized, the blood donor shortage would be solved in the blink of an eye!

Take-Home Messages

- Early diagnosis and treatment are key. We call this the "strike now before the iron gets too hot" strategy!
- The patient and his sister will have a full life despite this genetic disorder.
- His uncle had developed cirrhosis of the liver with complications, and these were treated with medicines. Despite removal of the excess iron by phlebotomy he unfortunately has a 25 to 30% chance of dying from primary cancer of the liver.
- Not everyone with the genetic mutation for hemochromatosis develops iron overload. Hence, we recommend that the test for the mutation only be done once there is documentation of iron overload by simple blood tests.

Non-Alcoholic Fatty Liver Disease (NAFLD)

Non-Alcoholic Liver Disease (NAFLD) is the most common chronic liver disease in the United States and the world. Recent estimates indicate that an alarming 70 to 100 million Americans are afflicted, and 1 billion have this condition worldwide. Yet, just a few decades ago, there was little or no mention of this liver disorder in medical textbooks. Its rise to epidemic levels has accompanied those of obesity and type 2 diabetes, and NAFLD is now rampant.

True to its name, when the liver tissue is examined under the microscope, the alterations in the liver cells are indistinguishable from those seen in alcoholic hepatitis, another common condition. However, these patients are typically drinking little or no alcohol.

Up to 70 % of patients with NAFLD also have type 2 diabetes. And most, but not all, people with NAFLD have metabolic syndrome, a cluster of conditions, including obesity, insulin resistance, high blood sugar, hypertension and high levels of fat (cholesterol and triglycerides) in the blood. In the United States, it is estimated that 50% of Americans over the age of 60 have metabolic syndrome. The contributing factors include a sedentary lifestyle, poor dietary habits, changes in the gut microbiome and hereditary factors.

NAFLD is a spectrum of diseases, ranging from increased fat deposition in the liver (fatty liver) to fat deposition and accompanying inflammation and liver damage (**non-alcoholic steatohepatitis (NASH)** to full-fledged cirrhosis. Most people with NAFLD have fatty liver, which is generally considered to be benign. However, about 15 to 20% of patients with NASH are estimated to progress to having cirrhosis. Once cirrhosis develops there is the potential for a host of life-threatening complications including liver failure, primary liver cancer and the need for a lifesaving liver transplantation. Indeed, in most centers in the United States NASH with cirrhosis and liver failure is the most common or second most common indication for liver transplantation.

> Some commonly used medications such as estrogens, steroids and tamoxifen can cause liver changes like those seen in patients with Non-Alcoholic Steatohepatitis (NASH), the more severe form of NAFLD.

The diagnosis of NAFLD is made on clinical grounds and the severity of disease can be assessed by either a liver biopsy or a special ultrasound of the liver, called a fibroscan. A fibroscan measures liver stiffness, which correlates with liver scarring (fibrosis). It is noninvasive, has gained acceptance and is becoming more readily available.

Note that a decade ago there were only a handful of NAFLD clinical trials running in the United States. At the time of this writing, there are now more than 425!

Recommendations: Managing NAFLD

- Your physician should check if you have antibodies protecting you from hepatitis A and B viruses. If not, vaccines are indicated.
- Coffee consumption is recommended. Patients with NASH who drink coffee have the least amount of fibrosis (scarring of the liver).
- If indicated, statins are safe to use and in fact may confer a reduction

in risk of developing primary liver cancer.

- The cornerstone of treatment is weight loss. We use motivational interviewing, support groups and different medicines to achieve this goal.
- Bariatric surgery for obesity can lead to reversal of diabetes and even reversal of early cirrhosis in a substantial number of patients.
- If you have NASH with or without cirrhosis, your clinician may wish to refer you to an academic center where clinical research on NASH is being conducted. As a patient, if eligible, you have the right to enroll in a clinical trial or to opt out without compromising your quality of care.

Key Points

- Patients with hemochromatosis who do not have diabetes or cirrhosis and are eligible for weekly phlebotomy to remove the excess iron in 18 months or less have the same life expectancy as individuals of the same gender and age who do not have hemochromatosis.
- Non-Alcoholic Liver Disease (NAFLD) is the dominant chronic liver disease in the United States and globally. Recent estimates indicate that an alarming 70 to 100 million Americans are afflicted with this condition, as are around 1 billion worldwide.
- Currently, the major treatment for NAFLD is weight loss. Given the plethora of clinical trials, it is very likely that other modalities of treatment will be available in the near future.

12

DIABETES AND GASTROINTESTINAL DISEASE

Now, good digestion wait on appetite, and health on both!

—William Shakespeare

The stomach and intestines can be adversely affected in several ways in people with diabetes to lead to bothersome symptoms. In this section we discuss gastroesophageal reflux disease, diabetic gastroparesis, diabetic diarrhea, emphysematous cholecystitis and the link between type 1 diabetes and celiac disease.

Gastroesophageal Reflux Disease (GERD)

Gastroesophageal reflux refers to the passage of contents in the stomach moving up into the esophagus. In healthy people without reflux, a ring-shaped sphincter muscle (the lower esophageal sphincter) between the esophagus and stomach prevents acidic contents in the stomach from entering the esophagus.

If this barrier is impaired, reflux can cause heartburn and, over time, can damage the lining of the esophagus leading to a narrowing (a stricture), bleeding and ulceration. In some severe cases, GERD can lead to a change in the lining called "Barrett's esophagus," which is associated with an increased risk of esophageal cancer.

People with diabetes are more prone to having an incompetent lower esophageal sphincter that, by not being able to close, allows reflux. Additionally, they are more likely to have a stomach that is slower to empty, what we call delayed gastric emptying, which can further aggravate the situation.

The most common symptom of GERD is heartburn. People may also experience chronic cough, hoarseness and a sense of shortness of breath often described as "asthma."

Management

Management includes the use of medications such as famotidine and omeprazole to decrease the stomach's secretion of gastric acid. Medications to enhance gastric emptying like metoclopramide are also useful.

Diabetic Gastroparesis

This is a syndrome characterized by nausea, vomiting, early satiety (a feeling of fullness soon after eating less than a full meal), bloating and abdominal discomfort or pain. In severe cases, it can cause weight loss.

Gastroparesis has been noted in 4 to 8% of people with type 1 diabetes and 1% of people with type 2 diabetes.

In 1958, Kassander coined the term "gastroparesis diabeticorum" to distinguish it from other causes of gastroparesis. Gastroparesis simply means that the stomach is not working efficiently as a pump to propel food out into the small intestine. In people with diabetes, it is believed to be caused by diabetic neuropathy (see page 67) of the nerves that control the stomach, slowing its reflexive muscular contractions.

> Medications used to control blood glucose such as GLP-1 receptor agonists (see page 154) should be avoided in people with gastroparesis and GERD, as they slow gastric emptying.

Management

Referral to a gastroenterologist for a definitive diagnosis and exclusion of an obstruction causing similar symptoms is recommended.

Management includes:

- Appropriate hydration, nutrition and blood sugar control.
- A diet low in both fat and in insoluble fiber.
- Some people are unable to tolerate solid food and need homogenized (liquified) foods for normal gastric emptying.
- Alcohol, smoking and carbonated beverages should be avoided.
- Medications such as metoclopramide, domperidone, cisapride and erythromycin can be used with success. Side effects may occur with these medications and patients must be educated about these.

Surgery for gastroparesis is only seldomly performed. One procedure involves electrical stimulation of the stomach to induce the stomach muscles to contract. The device runs on a battery that can last up to ten years. We recommend referral to an academic medical center if surgery is being contemplated.

Diabetic Diarrhea

Chronic diarrhea occurs in up to 20% of people with type 2 diabetes. The diarrhea seen in people with diabetes tends to be painless, non-bloody and can occur at night. Less frequently, people can also suffer from fecal incontinence.

Functional impairment of the nervous system of the gut, such as that caused by diabetic neuropathy (see page 67), can result in disordered motility of both the small and large intestine. This can lead to increased fluid secretion, as well as increased growth of bacteria in the small bowel (dysbiosis). Both neuropathy and intestinal dysbiosis can contribute to the occurrence of diarrhea in people with diabetes.

Diarrhea can also be caused by medications, such as metformin, or from ingesting artificial sweeteners, which may contain sorbitol. We often see this as a result of patients consuming so-called "dietetic" gum or candy!

Management

Management consists of medications that slow down the transit of stool in the gut, such as loperamide, and antispasmodic medications that reduce the frequency of bowel movements, such as bromide products.

Celiac Disease in Type 1 Diabetes

There is a well-documented association of type 1 diabetes and celiac disease, and 3 to 10% of people with type 1 diabetes have it. Individuals with celiac disease are intolerant of gluten, a protein present in wheat, barley, and rye.

Celiac disease can manifest in different ways, including diarrhea, unexplained iron deficiency anemia, or abnormal liver function tests. Management consists of following a gluten-free diet. Referral to a nutritionist for advice is of paramount importance, as avoiding gluten requires some work with research and adjustments in shopping and diet. It is in some surprising products, including instant coffee and even many medications!

Gallstones

Gallstones are solid deposits of components of digestive fluid that accumulate in the gallbladder. The two main types consist of cholesterol or pigment.

People with type 2 diabetes are more likely to develop cholesterol gallstones compared to individuals without diabetes. This increased risk is thought to be due to a higher amount of cholesterol present in the bile coming out of the liver. When this super-saturated bile is stored in the gallbladder, small cholesterol stones can form. Additionally, people with diabetes have less effective gallbladder emptying (into the small intestine), allowing stones more time to form.

In people with symptomatic gallstones - classically presenting with sudden pain in the right upper part of the abdomen or in the middle, above the belly button, and nausea or vomiting - the recommended treatment is removal of the gallbladder (**cholecystectomy**), most often performed laparoscopically.

Emphysematous Cholecystitis

This is a serious medical condition of infection of the gallbladder with gas-forming bacteria.

Affected patients are more often men, in the 40 to 70-year age range, and 30 to 50% of them have diabetes. Gangrene and perforation of the gallbladder can occur. Treatment consists of broad-spectrum antibiotics and urgent surgery to remove the gallbladder.

Patient Stories: A 62-Year-Old with New Onset Diarrhea

Ms. CD is a 62-year-old professor of history at a college in New England. She has had type 2 diabetes for three years and was started on metformin soon after the diagnosis was made. Her glucose control on metformin, together with diet and exercise, has been very good, and her most recent HbA1c was 6.4%.

At a follow-up appointment she told her physician that for the past two months she had experienced intermittent episodes of diarrhea which, she explained, as having three or four loose, watery stools. There was no blood in the stools, weight loss or incontinence.

Possible causes of diarrhea in people with diabetes:

1. Abnormal motility of the small and large bowel.
2. Increased intestinal secretions.
3. Bacterial overgrowth (dysbiosis).
4. Coexistence of celiac disease in people with type 1 diabetes.
5. Dietetic foods – e.g., candy, gum, drinks – containing sorbitol.
6. Medications – e.g., metformin, GLP-1 receptor agonists, Alpha-glucosidase inhibitors.

The endocrinologist discussed with the patient that the diarrhea could be secondary to metformin, even though she had been taking it for more than two years. The plan was to discontinue the metformin and see if the diarrhea resolved, rather than initiate a thorough and comprehensive evaluation.

The patient was asked to call to report progress a few weeks later. She did so and stated that her diarrhea had resolved completely within a week of stopping the metformin!

Take-Home Message

Approximately 5% of people who start metformin develop diarrhea, which is usually mild and transient. However, on rare occasions people taking it can develop diarrhea years after they have been on this medication. This was the cause of diarrhea in our patient. It is recommended that metformin be discontinued to see if the diarrhea abates, and only if it does not, to embark on a more comprehensive evaluation. Metformin can sometimes be restarted months later with no recurrence of the problem.

Key Points

- Gastroparesis has been noted in 4 to 8% of people with type 1 diabetes and 1% of people with type 2 diabetes.
- Chronic diarrhea occurs in up to 20% of people with type 2 diabetes. People can also have diarrhea secondary to medications (e.g., metformin) or from ingesting artificial sweeteners, which may contain sorbitol.
- There is a well-documented association of type 1 diabetes and celiac disease, and 3 to 10% of people with type 1 diabetes have it. Individuals with celiac disease are intolerant of gluten which is present in wheat, barley, and rye. Gluten is present in many foods, including instant coffee and is even an ingredient in many medications.

13

OTHER COMMON ISSUES AFFECTING PEOPLE WITH DIABETES

Be careful about reading health books. You may die of a misprint.

—Mark Twain

People with diabetes may experience many other medical conditions that can affect the quality of their lives and may also be disabling. These conditions are not unique to individuals with diabetes, but their recognition and management is paramount. Clinicians are usually aware of these disorders and work with the patient and their families to address them.

Eating Disorders

People, more often girls, with type 1 diabetes, are more prone to develop eating disorders. These range from fasting, self-induced vomiting, binging, and deliberately omitting or taking less than the prescribed dose of insulin, often referred to as **diabulimia**. People with eating disorders are more likely to develop complications and need more frequent hospitalization.

There is a useful screening tool that should be used particularly in adolescents and young adults to identify people with this problem – the Diabetes Eating Problems Survey-Revised. At some diabetes centers a comprehensive team approach has been implemented to address this challenge.

Sleep Disorders

Both quantity and quality of sleep have been shown to be an independent risk factor for the development of type 2 diabetes.

In a meta-analysis of 10 prospective studies by Cappuccio and colleagues published in *Diabetes Care* in 2010, it was noted that the quantity and quality of sleep was shown to be an independent risk factor for the development of type 2 diabetes. People who lacked enough sleep were more likely to develop chronic illnesses including type 2 diabetes.

Sleep apnea is a very common condition and occurs in both obese and non-obese individuals. It is also more prevalent in people with type 2 diabetes. It has been shown that effective treatment for sleep apnea, such as continuous positive airways pressure (CPAP), improves glucose control. This was documented by Malik and colleagues in the *Indian Journal of Endocrinology and Metabolism* in 2017.

Common Medications That Can Increase Blood Glucose Levels

There are many commonly used medications that can increase blood glucose levels.

Statins

Statins are a common class of drugs used to lower cholesterol levels and reduce the risk for coronary artery disease and stroke. They are extremely well-tolerated in general, but several recent studies have drawn attention to the fact that they may increase blood glucose levels. There is a dose-dependent effect, meaning that the higher the dose of statin, the greater the increase in blood glucose levels. The increase, however, is very modest and all experts agree that the benefits of statin therapy outweigh this side effect.

In an article in the *Lancet* in 2012, Ridker and colleagues concluded that, "the cardiovascular and mortality benefits of statin therapy exceed the diabetes hazard, including in participants at high risk of developing diabetes."

Antipsychotic Medications

Antipsychotic medications have been shown to be associated with weight gain, diabetes and abnormal blood lipid levels (referred to as part of metabolic syndrome).

These drugs are of significant clinical utility and should be continued if appropriate. The magnitude of these side effects varies amongst the many antipsychotic drugs in current use. Your primary care clinician or psychiatrist can safely guide you. Sometimes switching from one medication to another may reduce these untoward side effects.

We recommend that patients taking these drugs be regularly monitored for weight gain and diabetes.

Thiazides

Thiazide drugs used to treat high blood pressure can sometimes increase blood glucose levels, but lower doses (currently preferred for treatment of hypertension) are much less likely to do so.

Glucocorticoids

Glucocorticoids (steroids), a commonly used medicine for a variety of conditions, are also known to increase blood glucose levels significantly. There is a dose-dependent effect, in other words, the higher the dose of the medicine, the greater the potential increase in blood glucose. Steroids given to people without diabetes on a long-term basis may cause a form of type 2 diabetes that we call **steroid-induced diabetes**. In most cases, it resolves soon after stopping steroids.

Musculoskeletal Problems

Musculoskeletal problems are often encountered in people with diabetes and can lead discomfort, pain and decreased mobility. Most are related to the slow cumulative damage to connective tissue and scarring (fibroproliferation) associated with diabetes.

Hand

Knots of tissue can accumulate in the palm of the hand. This is called **Dupuytren's contracture** and can lead to one or more fingers being bent – called "trigger fingers." This can interfere with grasping a golf club or tennis racquet. Dupuytren's contracture is also seen in other medical disorders, such as due to alcoholism. If necessary, this can be treated with a steroid injection or surgical release.

Cheiroarthropathy ("diabetic stiff hand syndrome") is seen in up to 50% of people with both type 1 and type 2 diabetes. It is caused by a thickening of the tissues under the skin and can limit the ability to hold the hands both flat on a table or in a "prayer pose," with palms held flat together. It does not usually lead to discomfort but is a useful physical sign for clinicians – one that can be assessed in a few seconds.

Wrist

Carpal tunnel syndrome is a common condition that is unfortunately even more frequent in people with diabetes compared to those without the condition. The median nerve – a major nerves of the wrist and hand – is compressed as it travels through a narrowing in the wrist. This leads to pain, numbness and tingling in the hand, sometimes extending to the arm.

It is also more common in in several other conditions, including rheumatoid arthritis, thyroid conditions and in people who use vibrating tools on a regular basis. It can be treated with simple splints, steroid injections and, sometimes, surgery.

Shoulder

Frozen shoulder is a condition that causes stiffness and pain in the shoulder joint. It is caused by thickening of the capsule that surrounds the tendons and ligaments of the shoulder joint. It is more common in people with diabetes but is also seen in several other conditions, such as after rotator cuff injury or in any condition associated with decreased movement of the shoulder. Treatment consists of physical therapy and injection of steroids into the joint. Rarely, arthroscopic surgery is necessary.

Rotator cuff syndrome is another common condition that occurs even more commonly in people with diabetes or in people with jobs or activities requiring repetitive overhead actions, such as tennis players, basketball athletes. Rotator cuff muscles maintain the stability of the shoulder joint. Treatment consists of rest, physical therapy, steroid injections and, occasionally, surgery.

Knee

Diabetes can be caused by excessive iron accumulation in the pancreas, as part of a common hereditary condition called **genetic hemochromatosis** (see page 82). People with this condition can present with severe pain and swelling in the knee. As a part of diagnosis, a sample of fluid from the knee joint is aspirated (removed) and examined under a microscope, revealing characteristic crystal formations. These crystals consist of calcium pyrophosphate and their presence in joints (most commonly the knee) is called **pseudogout**.

In "normal" gout, the crystals consist of uric acid and most commonly affect the big toe. Pseudogout can be seen in other conditions such as an underactive thyroid gland or an overactive parathyroid gland. These conditions need to be ruled out in someone who presents with pseudogout.

Sexual Dysfunction in Diabetes

Sexual dysfunction - an inability to experience satisfactory sexual activity - can be seen in both men and women with diabetes. It can be encountered in people with both type 1 and type 2 diabetes. It appears to be more prevalent in men, and the commonest symptom is **erectile dysfunction**.

Individuals with long-standing diabetes, especially if they have other complications, such as neuropathy, retinopathy, and cardiovascular disease, are more likely to have sexual dysfunction. Approximately 50% of such individuals will have symptoms. There are very effective treatments for this condition.

Less is known about the prevalence and nature of sexual dysfunction in women with diabetes. Issues include low libido, vaginal dryness, difficulty achieving an orgasm as well as an increased incidence of urinary tract infections (UTIs). Psychosexual issues appear to be more common in those with co-existent depression.

Mental Health Challenges in People with Diabetes

People with diabetes face many challenges every day of their lives. These include watching what they eat, finding the motivation to exercise, taking many medications (oral or injectable), testing their blood glucoses frequently, and seeing many different health care providers frequently. Not surprisingly, those with diabetes are two to three times more likely to suffer from **depression** than people without diabetes.

Symptoms of depression can vary from being mild to severe. These may include:

- Losing interest in previously enjoyable activities or hobbies.

- Feeling fatigued for most of the day.
- Having difficulty focusing and making decisions.
- Change in appetite – either eating too much or too little.
- Not being able to have a good night's sleep.
- Feeling helpless and hopeless.
- Having thoughts of suicide or death.

Sadly, less than 50% of people with diabetes who have depression are accurately diagnosed and treated. Importantly, treatment – including medications, psychotherapy, meditation, and exercise – is usually very effective and improves quality of life significantly.

The constellation of the many challenges people with diabetes face daily can lead to a feeling of being overwhelmed and distraught. This has been referred to as **diabetes distress** or burnout. It is incumbent for anyone with diabetes who is experiencing these feelings to seek professional help right away.

'Diabetes distress' is the feeling of being overwhelmed and distraught due to the many daily challenges people with diabetes face. Don't forget, there are many people in the same position and there are effective therapies you can try!

Brittle Diabetes

Brittle, or labile, diabetes is a term that was previously used in people with type 1 diabetes to describe wide swings in blood glucose, but it is seldomly used today in clinical practice. In many instances, the wide fluctuations in blood glucose are due to poor management of diet and/or use of insulin.

Clinicians should rule out celiac disease or other disorders of nutrient absorption when encountering such individuals.

Diabetes and COVID-19 infection

There is no evidence that having diabetes increases susceptibility to acquiring COVID-19 infection. There is evidence, however, that people with diabetes who acquire COVID-19 may have a more severe form of the infection. This is because patients with poorly controlled diabetes and high glucose levels have an impaired ability to fight any type of infection, due to an impaired function of white blood cells, the "soldiers" that defend the body against pathogenic microbes. They have an increased risk of mortality as compared to people with well-controlled diabetes, whose risk of mortality is much lower.

Surgery and Diabetes

People with diabetes often undergo surgery - ambulatory or in hospital surgery - such as a total knee or hip replacement or cardiac surgery, to name a few procedures. Management of blood glucose levels and optimal blood pressure control is critical in minimizing the risk of complications, particularly serious infections.

Surgery is often stressful. Anesthesia, surgery and trauma can all contribute to a marked increase in the stress hormones cortisol and catecholamines, which raise the blood sugar levels. This in turn, can lead to:

- **Sepsis**: a serious infection in tissues, organs and the blood).
- **Ischemia** (decreased blood flow) to the brain.
- **Impaired wound healing**.
- Some anesthetic and sedation **medications** may also adversely affect blood sugar levels.

On the other hand, hypoglycemia can also occur. This can lead to dire consequences including the development of coma and seizures. This prolongs the duration of hospitalization, increases the need for admission to an intensive care unit (ICU), and increases the risk of mortality.

Thus, appropriate management is needed before, during and after surgery (often referred to as the **perioperative period**) to ensure good outcomes.

Recommendations: Preparing for Surgery

We offer some guidelines below. Please note that this does **not** substitute for expert management by your primary care clinician, surgery team, hospitalist, or if necessary, your endocrinologist.

1. If you smoke or drink alcohol, it is best to stop or markedly curtail these habits for at least two weeks before any elective surgery.
2. If you are able, perform 20 to 30 minutes of aerobic exercise daily for at least two weeks before surgery.

3. Monitor your blood glucose levels frequently and, if necessary, adjust the dose of the medications you are taking.
4. Certain medicines need to be discontinued before surgery. For example, in the US and Europe, metformin is discontinued immediately prior to surgery due to the potential risk of kidney complications that can occur during or following surgery. Many other medicines are also often stopped prior to surgery because they can alter gastric emptying, which might increase the risk for nausea or vomiting in the postoperative period. Some medications may also have deleterious effects on blood sugar levels.
5. Studies suggest that patients who have blood sugar levels of 140 to 170 mg/dL [7.8–9.4 mmol/L] during surgery have the lowest risk of adverse outcomes.
6. After an operation, blood sugar levels between 140 and 180 mg/dL [7.8–10 mmol/L] are felt to be optimal and recommended by the American Diabetes Association, the American Association of Clinical Endocrinologists and the American Society of Thoracic Surgeons.
7. Insulin requirements are generally higher in patients undergoing cardiac surgery and tight glucose control in these patients leads to improved outcomes.
8. Ideally, all people with diabetes, particularly those on insulin regimens, should undergo elective surgery prior to 9 am to minimize disruption of their usual schedule.

Key Points

- Recent studies have drawn attention to the fact that statins may increase blood glucose levels. There is a dose-dependent effect, meaning that the higher the dose of statin the greater the increase in blood glucose levels. The increase, however, is very modest and all experts agree that the benefits of statin therapy outweigh this side effect.
- Anesthesia, surgery and trauma can markedly increase stress hormones such as cortisol and catecholamines, which raise blood sugar levels. This can lead to serious complications such as sepsis, decreased blood flow to the brain, and slowed wound healing.

14

DIET

I will use those dietary regimens which will benefit my patients according to my greatest ability and judgement, and I will do no harm or injustice to them.

—Hippocratic Oath (excerpt)

Some questions we are regularly asked by people who have been diagnosed with prediabetes or diabetes are, "What can I eat?"; "Is there a special diet that will help?"; "How much weight should I lose?"; and "Is it better for me to have diet sodas as opposed to regular sodas?"

It is no surprise that some of the most popular internet searches that patients conduct regarding the management of their diabetes relate to food.

In this chapter we discuss some of the specific types of dietary interventions that have been studied in people with type 2 diabetes or prediabetes. Let's begin by addressing some seminal facts that arose from landmark studies.

The Evidence

A landmark trial called the Diabetes Prevention Program was designed to compare a lifestyle intervention program with no specific intervention or medications in people who had prediabetes and were overweight or obese. Those who were randomized to participate in the lifestyle intervention component of the study lost approximately 7% of their body weight and in doing so reduced the risk for the progression to type 2 diabetes by a staggering 58%! This outcome was superior to that seen in people who were randomized to take the glucose lowering medication metformin. Their risk reduction was 30%. Studies like this done in other parts of the world have yielded identical results (see page 29).

In another study called Look AHEAD (Action for Health in Diabetes) conducted in people with type 2 diabetes, people in the lifestyle intervention were more likely to achieve complete or partial remission of their diabetes compared with the education and support group, who just received some advice but were not actively involved in lifestyle intervention.

The lifestyle intervention in the above studies comprised a reduced calorie diet (low-fat) and moderately intense exercise (walking briskly for 30 minutes, five times a week).

What we have gleaned from these studies is that, for individuals who have diabetes and are overweight or obese, a small amount of weight loss (5 to 10% of body weight) can make a major difference in lowering glucose (HbA1c), **and** in lowering blood pressure **and** serum cholesterol (the so-called "ABCs" of diabetes management – HbA1c, blood pressure and cholesterol). In those with nona-alcoholic fatty liver disease (NAFLD; see page 85) a similar degree of weight loss also has a significant benefit and is currently the cornerstone of therapy.

Is there one diet that is better than all others? This is the million-dollar question!

The evidence thus far suggests that one type of diet is not necessarily better than another. What is important if you need to lose weight is your ability to adhere to a dietary plan and maintain weight loss. Many different types of diets can result in weight loss, improved glucose control, and sometimes even remission of diabetes if enough weight is lost and the weight is kept off. There are at least half a dozen "diets" for which there are peer reviewed publications in reputable journals. This is what we know so far....

> The key factor in choosing a weight loss diet is your ability to **adhere** to a dietary plan and **maintain** weight loss.

The Mediterranean Diet

With the observation that coronary heart disease was less prevalent and hence caused fewer deaths in Mediterranean countries, such as Italy and Greece, compared to Northern Europe and the United Sates, researchers wondered whether it had something to do with the diet consumed in these countries.

Early studies demonstrated that the Mediterranean diet is associated with fewer risk factors for coronary heart disease. Indeed, the data is so impressive that the Mediterranean diet is recommended as a healthy eating plan in the dietary guidelines for Americans to promote health and prevent chronic disease. It is also endorsed by the World Health Organization.

There is no single definition of what the Mediterranean diet is, but it is high in vegetables, fruits, whole grains, beans, nut and seeds, and olive oil.

Major recommendations are:

- Have vegetables, fruits, healthy fats and whole grains every day. Olive oil is an example of a healthy fat, and its use is encouraged.
- Eat fish, poultry, eggs (less than 4 per week) and beans every week.
- Dairy products, such as yoghurt and cheese, should be consumed in moderate amounts.
- Limit your intake of red meat.

Other tangible elements of the Mediterranean diet include the social connectedness that comes from sharing meals with family and friends, enjoying a glass of red wine, maintaining an active lifestyle, and possibly more sunny days which would translate into higher vitamin levels!

> Fatty fish, such as sardines, mackerel, salmon, albacore tuna and lake trout are excellent sources of **omega-3 fatty acids**. These essential nutrients have been shown to lower blood pressure and triglycerides, slow the development of plaque in arteries and reduce the risk of heart attacks, strokes and sudden cardiac death.

The Evidence

The Mediterranean diet has been shown to reduce the risk of developing diabetes, lower HbA1c in people with type 2 diabetes, promote weight loss, and reduce the risk of major cardiovascular events. It has also been shown to increase telomere length. **Telomeres** are caps at the end of chromosomes analogous to the plastic tip at the end of our shoelaces. They prevent both fraying of chromosomes and prevent the chromosomes from sticking to each other. Telomere length is linked to cellular ageing and those with increased length are believed to have a longer life expectancy. Elizabeth Blackburn, a brilliant Australian scientist, and two colleagues received the Nobel prize in Medicine or Physiology in 2009 for their seminal work on telomeres.

Low- or Very Low-Fat Diet

In the mid to late 1970s the American Heart Association and the United States government started urging Americans to limit the amount of fat they consumed in their diet in the hope that it would lower blood cholesterol levels and hence the risk of cardiovascular disease.

However, the scientific evidence that limiting dietary fat lowered the risk of atherosclerosis was weak and the recommendation was dropped in 2010. We now know that there are "good fats" and "bad fats." Examples of good fats include monounsaturated and polyunsaturated fats, such those found in fish, nuts and olive oil. And examples of bad fats include saturated fats such as those from animal fats, and trans fats.

Therefore, this diet encourages individuals to consume vegetables, fruits, starches (bread, pasta, whole grains, starchy vegetables), lean protein, and low-fat dairy products. The percentage of calories derived from fats range from 10% (very low-fat) to 30% (low-fat). Based on the above information, anyone following this diet should avoid "bad fats." Remember that some vitamins are fat soluble. These include vitamins A, D, E, and K. Hence, if you are not consuming enough dietary fat, you could become deficient in these vitamins, leading to serious health consequences.

The Evidence

Adherence to these diets results in weight loss, and reduced risk for development of diabetes. Additionally, the very low-fat diet also leads to a lowering of blood pressure.

Low- and Very Low-Carbohydrate Diets

Low-carbohydrate (low-carb) diets limit carbohydrates, such as those found in grains, starchy vegetables, and fruit, and emphasize foods that are high in protein and fat. There are many types and variations of low-carb diets. Each diet has varying restrictions on the types and amounts of carbohydrates you can eat.

A low-carb diet restricts the type and amount of carbohydrates you eat. Carbohydrates can be simple or complex. Simple carbohydrates include refined sugar, and foods containing white flour. Complex carbohydrates include whole grains and beans

As the name implies, a low-carb diet limits the amount of carbohydrates and in turn, emphasizes the consumption of proteins, which include meat, poultry, fish, eggs, cheese, nuts and seeds.

These diets also incorporate the use of vegetables low in carbohydrate, such as salad greens, broccoli, cauliflower, cucumber, cabbage and mushrooms; fat from animal foods, oils, butter, and avocado. Starchy and sugary foods such as pasta, rice, potatoes, bread, and sweets are restricted. A low-carbohydrate diet has anywhere between 25 and 45% of calories as carbohydrate; a very low-carbohydrate diet limits the amount of carbohydrate further to less than 25% of total calories.

A very low-carbohydrate diet may lead to nutritional ketosis (increased production of ketones which the body uses as an alternate source of energy) - this is called a "**keto diet**."

> A "keto diet" is a very low-carbohydrate diet that can lead to nutritional ketosis – increased production of ketones, an alternate energy source.

The Evidence

These diets have been shown to promote weight loss, lower HbA1c, lower blood pressure and improve lipid profiles.

The Atkins Diet

A popular diet that many people are familiar with is called the Atkins diet. This is named after Robert C. Atkins, a physician who popularized it in the 1960s. Dr. Atkins believed that fats should not be limited, that the fat in fatty meats should not be trimmed off, and that these fats were in fact healthy to eat. He felt that carbohydrates were "the real enemy," in that they caused marked increases in glucose which led to the release of insulin, which in turn promoted fat deposition in the body.

The Evidence

A common claim is that one can lose 15 pounds [6.8 kg] in the first two weeks of this diet. However, the studies looking at long-term health outcomes are lacking. Many physicians believe that eating a large amount of fats and animal protein will likely increase the risk of cardiovascular disease and even certain cancers.

The South Beach Diet

This is another weight-loss diet created in 2003 by cardiologist Arthur Agatston, MD, and it gained popularity after publication of his best-selling book "The South Beach Diet: The Delicious, Doctor-Designed, Foolproof Plan for Fast and Healthy Weight Loss."

It is sometimes called a modified low-carbohydrate diet because it is not a strict low-carb diet.

There is also a keto (ketogenic) version of the South Beach diet, which allows for very few carbohydrates. The goal of a ketogenic diet is to force the body to use fat rather than carbohydrates or protein as the main source of energy.

The South Beach Diet also limits unhealthy fats and encourages the consumption of more fiber, whole grains, fruits and vegetables.

The Evidence

The claims are that people who go on this diet lose 8 to 13 pounds [3.6-5.9 kg] in the first two weeks. Long-term outcome studies are not known. However, consumption of food that is rich in healthy carbohydrates and healthy fats can improve one's health and may improve cholesterol levels. It is generally considered to be a safe diet.

The DASH Diet

This Dietary Approaches to Stop Hypertension (DASH) diet encourages vegetables, fruits, low-fat dairy products, whole grains, poultry, fish, and nuts. It limits red meat, sugary products and sodium. It was originally developed for the treatment of hypertension.

The Evidence

Adherence to this diet leads to a reduced risk of developing diabetes. It also promotes weight loss and lowers blood pressure.

Vegetarian or Vegan Diet

These diets are devoid of all flesh foods. Eggs are permitted in the vegetarian diet. The vegan diet is more restrictive and eggs and dairy products are not allowed.

The Evidence

These diets have been shown to reduce the risk of developing diabetes, lower HbA1c in individuals with diabetes, promote weight loss and to improve the lipid profile.

Strict adherence to vegan and plant-based diets has been shown to reverse coronary atherosclerosis, as documented by coronary angiography.

Paleo Diet

A paleo diet is essentially consuming foods that are similar to what we think was consumed during the paleolithic era (2.5 million to 10,000 years ago). Other names include the stone age diet, the paleolithic diet, the caveman diet and the hunter-gatherer diet.

This diet is based on the food man could obtain by hunting and gathering. Thus, it typically includes lean meats, fish, fruits, vegetables, nuts, and seeds. This diet had minimal amounts of dairy products, legumes and grains.

The Evidence

Several clinical trials have shown that the benefits of paleo include:

- Better appetite management.
- Weight loss.
- Improved glucose tolerance.
- Improved blood pressure control.
- Lower triglycerides.

There are no long-term studies addressing the health benefits of the paleo diet. We conclude that it may help you lose weight or maintain a steady weight. But because this diet does not include whole grains and legumes and therefore is low in fiber and some vitamins, we recommend supplementing the diet with fiber and vitamins, and discussing this with your nutritionist.

Long-term Adherence

Of all the different types of dietary interventions, the Mediterranean diet is the one that has been studied the most and has been shown to improve glucose control, facilitate weight loss, and reduce cardiovascular risk.

The key to success is long-term adherence to a diet that you can maintain and enables you to achieve the goals that you and your clinician have established.

Glycemic Index

Many readers will be familiar to some extent with these terms. Permit us to elaborate and explain in simple terms.

The glycemic index (GI) refers to a system of assigning a number to carbohydrate-containing foods based on how much it increases blood sugar. The number is derived from comparing the ingestion of 50 grams of the food with a reference food, usually white bread. Foods with a higher GI cause a greater rise in blood glucose levels. It is an invaluable tool in guiding food choices.

There are three categories:

1. **Low GI**: 55 or less.
2. **Medium GI**: 56 to 69.
3. **High GI**: 70 or more.

Glycemic Load

Glycemic load (GL) incorporates both the GI and the amount of the food eaten in a serving and is therefore a better estimate of the amount of glucose that will enter the blood. An illustrative example is watermelon. This has a high GI but since a typical serving does not contain many carbohydrates, the GL is low.

In a meta-analysis of six trials (totaling 202 participants), both short-term weight loss and a reduction in LDL cholesterol were evident. However, there have so far been no trials lasting more than six months, so the long-term benefits are unknown.

The complete list of the GI and GL for more than 1,000 foods can be found in the article "International Tables Of Glycemic Index And Glycemic Load Values: 2008" by Fiona S. Atkinson and colleagues, which was published in the journal *Diabetes Care* that same year.

Foods with a high glycemic index not only affect blood sugar levels, but also have an impact on cardiovascular disease and mortality. In a seminal study published in the *New England Journal of Medicine* in 2021, David Jenkins et al. detail the results of an analysis of more than

The Glycemic Index (GI) of Some Common Foods

Low GI	Medium GI	High GI
Green vegetables	Brown rice	White rice
Raw carrots	Sweet corn	White bread
Chickpeas	Bananas	Potatoes, including mashed potatoes that are peeled and boiled
Lentils	Raw pineapple	
Most fruits	Multigrain, oat bran, rye bread	
Bran breakfast cereals	Oat-based breakfast cereals	
Sweet potatoes (unpeeled)		

130,000 participants from 20 countries in five continents. They concluded that people who consumed foods with a high glycemic index had a significant increase in risk for developing cardiovascular disease and death from cardiovascular disease.

> If you reduce caloric intake by 500 calories per day (3500 calories in a week) it is likely that you will lose 1 pound per week.

Intermittent Fasting

For thousands of years, fasting was considered a form of medicine. Many of the revered doctors of ancient times recommended fasting as a critically important component of both prevention and healing. Ayurvedic medicine, with a history of 5,000 years, also advocates fasting as an important treatment. None other than Hippocrates, who is considered the father of Western medicine, believed that fasting allowed the body to heal itself.

The Evidence

Studies in animal models have consistently found that intermittent fasting has major benefits in a wide range of chronic disorders, including diabetes, obesity, cardiovascular disease, cancers, and neurodegenerative brain diseases. Fasting enables the body to utilize ketones rather than carbohydrates as the fuel required for energy production.

Two general ways that it appears to improve health at a cellular level are by triggering alternative pathways that can better cope with stress on the cell and counteract some disease processes, and by protecting DNA from damage and increasing the "culling" of damaged cells (by "apoptosis," programmed cell death, essentially a cell suicide mechanism), such as may be operative in many cancers.

> Studies in animals have consistently found that intermittent fasting has major benefits in a many chronic disorders, including diabetes, obesity, cardiovascular disease, cancers, and neurodegenerative brain diseases.

There may be other mechanisms involved, including alteration of the gut microbiome to a less proinflammatory profile.

What do the human studies reveal? Intermittent fasting has been shown to have benefits for a broad range of common health conditions, including diabetes, obesity, cardiovascular disease, cancers and neurological disorders. What remains to be seen is whether this can be adopted by millions and millions of people worldwide and maintained for years. In many different animal species caloric deprivation leads to a significantly longer lifespan. Whether this will happen in humans needs to be determined.

A study published in the journal *Cell Metabolism* in July 2020, shed more light on this subject. The researchers randomly assigned 58 obese men and women to three groups. The first group were only allowed to eat between 3 pm and 7 pm, while the second group could only eat between 1 pm and 7 pm. The third group ate whenever they wanted. None of the participants were told to restrict caloric intake.

In the two groups that practiced time-restricted fasting, participants consumed an average of 550 fewer calories a day and lost about 3% of their body weight over the 8-week study period. Furthermore, those in the time-restricted fasting groups demonstrated reductions in both fasting insulin and insulin resistance, which could imply a reduced risk for diabetes.

"Our main finding here is that time-restricted fasting cuts out 550 calories a day, which is very hard to do in an ordinary calorie-restricted diet," said the senior author, Krista Varady, a professor of nutrition at the University of Illinois, Chicago. "The coolest part is that it's so simple. All you have to do is watch the clock."

For more about this topic, we recommend an elegant and very

comprehensive 2019 review from by de Cabo and Mattson in the *New England Journal of Medicine*.

Approaches

There are various approaches to practice intermittent fasting. A popular and easy one is the "sixteen-hour fast." This means that if you finish eating dinner at 7 pm, your next meal would not be before 11 am the following morning. What helps enormously is that for much of that time you are sleeping! Then, in the morning, only non-caloric beverages area allowed: coffee, tea, and water. Hence, all your caloric consumption occurs between 11 am and 7 pm.

Of note, there are no recommendations as to which foods should be consumed and which should be avoided. Many people tell us that they do not feel hungry during this sixteen-hour period and in fact feel more energized. One of the authors of this book has done this and can attest to this experience.

There are other more severe approaches to fasting, such as fasting for two or even three days of the week.

Weight Status

We use the body mass index (BMI) to determine weight status. It is calculated as weight in kg divided by height (in m^2). The optimal BMI is between 19 and 24.9 kg/m^2. Overweight is defined as a BMI of 25 or more and obesity as 30 or more.

In people of Asian origin, a BMI of 23 or greater is considered overweight.

Recommendations: Planning Your Diet

There is no "one size fits all" diet but, regardless of how it is achieved, **sustained** weight loss leads to remarkable benefits. These include reduction in medication requirements and, occasionally, even remission of type 2 diabetes!

As you are doubtlessly aware, there are three main macronutrients in our diet: carbohydrates, proteins and fats.

> Regardless of how it is achieved, weight loss, if sustained, leads to remarkable benefits. These include reduction in medication requirements and, occasionally, even remission of type 2 diabetes.

There is no ideal amount of each that should be prescribed for individuals with diabetes or prediabetes, just as there is no specific "diet" that will be universally successful. It is important to individualize dietary recommendations based on the current eating habits, ability to change eating habits, and the goals of therapy.

There are, however, basic recommendations that apply to everyone:

- Intake of dietary **fiber** should be increased and should be a minimum of 14 grams per 1000 calories per day. This is best achieved by eating foods that have lots of fiber, e.g., non-starchy vegetables, fruits, whole grains. Sometimes dietary supplements are needed. Adding more fiber alone to the diet can facilitate some weight loss and improvement in glucose control.
- **Carbohydrates** rich in fiber, vitamins and minerals and low in sugars and fats are encouraged. This once again includes whole grains, fruits, vegetables, legumes and low-fat milk. We sometimes use the glycemic index to identify which carbohydrates are preferable (remember that there may be individual variations in blood glucose rise following ingestion of the same food). In general, people with diabetes should aim to reduce their carbohydrate intake, as this has been shown to have the best impact on glucose levels. For some people, low-carbohydrate or very low-carbohydrate diets may be very helpful and may help improve glucose control where other dietary interventions have not succeeded.
- **Proteins** derived from plants, fish and poultry are generally preferred to animal-derived proteins. Lean meats, fish, eggs, beans, peas, nuts, soy products and seeds are preferable to red meat. The type of protein should be lean protein more than protein that contains a saturated fat.
- **Fat**: The type of fat eaten is also extremely important; mono- and polyunsaturated fats are far healthier than saturated fats. Saturated fats derived from animal products, such as red meat, are discouraged, whereas foods like fish, olive oil and nuts and some vegetables like avocados are encouraged.
- **Dairy**: Ingestion of at least two servings of dairy products (milk, cheese, yoghurt) has been shown to reduce the risk for development of diabetes, hypertension, and other factors for development of heart disease. This study included thousands of individuals from multiple countries and was published by Bhavadharini and

colleagues in 2020.

- **Vitamin D** supplementation has been shown in one study to reduce the risk for the development of type 2 diabetes in people with prediabetes. This was shown in large multi-center study called the "Vitamin D and Type 2 Diabetes Study" conducted in the United States.
- **Fruit**: Increased consumption of fruit lowers the risk for developing type 2 diabetes. In contrast, increased consumption of fruit juices increases the risk.
- The addition of **cinnamon** may prevent progression from prediabetes to diabetes in some individuals. The data supporting this is preliminary and needs to be validated.

Type 1 Diabetes

For people with type 1 diabetes, the above general principles apply. It is important to ensure that there is either consistent carbohydrate intake which is covered with an appropriate dose of insulin at each meal, or that people learn to count carbohydrates and administer their insulin based on the amount of carbohydrate eaten at the meal.

We encourage people with type 1 diabetes to learn advanced carbohydrate counting - this enables people to adjust the dose of insulin based on the amount of carbohydrate eaten and their glucose level prior to the meal.

Foods that have a low GI and GL will cause less excessive rises in glucose than more "sugary" products and these are thus preferred to higher GI carbohydrates.

Understanding the Evidence and Choosing a Diet

There are many publications in the medical literature spouting the benefits of different diets in people with type 2 diabetes. They range from case reports to non-randomized studies and a few studies comparing one dietary intervention with another. For example, there are case reports of three people with type 2 diabetes who were able to stop insulin after starting an intermittent fasting program. It is not clear if they could stop their other medications for diabetes.

There are non-randomized studies of hundreds of people with type 2 diabetes who followed a low-carbohydrate/keto diet that included

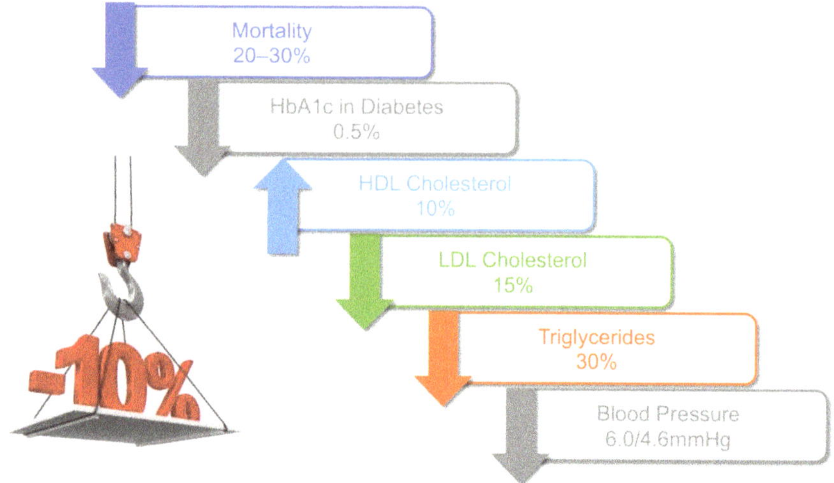

A loss of 5-10% body weight has impressive benefits! Adapted from the ASCEND (Academy for Science and Continuing Education in Diabetes and Obesity) Program. http://www.ASCEND-diabetes-obesity.com.

remote monitoring and who were followed for one year. The results? A marked reduction in HbA1c, almost 50% of the participants stopped their insulin and almost two thirds of stopped their diabetes medications altogether! There is also a controlled study comparing the Mediterranean diet with a low-carb diet, which showed that after 1 year there really was no difference in the amount of weight lost. And so, unfortunately, there are no long-term studies showing that one diet is better than another.

In medicine, we often see pilot studies with only a few patients that present spectacular results, only to later be disappointed with the results of more rigorous studies. Sir William Osler once said, "The best time to use a new drug is right away while it's still working." We paraphrase this: "The best time to use a new diet is right away, while it's still working!"

We encourage people with diabetes to seek the advice of a **nutritionist** for nutrition counseling. "Medical nutrition therapy" provides an opportunity for people with diabetes to be counselled about weight management, physical activity, caloric intake, and education about meal planning.

What's the bottom line? If you need to lose weight and are going to embark on a particular "diet," choose one that you will be able to adhere to long-term. Most important of all, when it comes to eating, make healthy choices - choose healthy carbohydrates, proteins, and fats, and make sure you have enough vitamins and minerals, too!

And eat your food slowly, chew it well and, ideally, enjoy the ritual with your family or friends!

Motivational Interviewing

Motivational interviewing is a technique that helps a clinician and patient work together to achieve a desired goal. It has been successfully employed to help people lose weight, exercise and stop smoking. The clinician prompts the patient using key questions. The answers by the patient clearly identify ways in which he or she can succeed in achieving that goal. To emphasize, the clinician is not telling or preaching to the patient what needs to be done.

The following conversation illustrates the principles of motivational interviewing:

- Clinician: "On a scale of 1 to 10, 1 being least important and 10 being critically important, how important is it for you to lose weight?"
- Patient: "Oh I would say a 9, maybe 10."
- Clinician: "On a scale of 1 to 10, one being easy and 10 being very, very difficult, how difficult is it to lose weight?"
- Patient: "A 10 .... maybe 11!"
- Clinician: "What could you do to cut down the calories you consume?"
- Patient: "Hmmm....well, I could have one toast instead of two with my breakfast? Or I could try adding only one spoon of sugar to my coffee. I have four cups a day. I could eat ice cream twice a week, not daily?"
- Clinician: "That might decrease your weekly caloric intake by 3500 calories or so. That equates to losing up to one pound per week. So, on a scale of 1 to 10....this time 10 being very, very easy, and 1 being very difficult, what do you think are the chances of achieving this?"
- Patient: "Probably an 8."
- Clinician: "Great! Let me see you in follow-up in two to three months. I hope to see you 8 to 12 pounds [3.6–5.4 kg] lighter!"

- Both clinician and patient smile.

This technique is useful in helping patients lose weight up to 50% of the time. Yet this whole process takes only three to four minutes! As an exercise, consider your own answers as the patient in the above conversation.

Patient TF's Story

> *I was diagnosed with diabetes right after I got out of the Navy, and I lived with diabetes for almost 2 decades. I'd had enough of being overweight, unable even to walk upstairs to go to bed without my knees hurting. I was taking all kinds of meds for my type 2 diabetes. Enough was enough!*

And so, Tim embarked on a weight loss diet coupled with online coaching:

> *My entire life has changed. My HbA1c went from 6.5 to 5.5, and I was able to go off of several medications. I started out at 328 pounds [149 kg] and now run around 220 [99.8 kg]. I've had to buy all new clothes. I had not been able to wear my Navy uniform to military functions. I'm happy to say that just last week I had a function that was full military honors—and guess what? I fit back into my uniform from 21 years ago!*

Patient KJ's Story

> *I started my weight loss program using a prescribed very low-carbohydrate diet coupled with ongoing healthy coaching. I started at 328 pounds with a waist size of 58 inches, and I am now 228 pounds with a 46-inch waist. I am off of 8 prescription meds, and I have lost 100 pounds [45.4 kg] and kept it off, all while healing my body.*
>
> *It has been two years of healing. Just today my fasting blood sugar was 125, and at the start of the program my fasting blood sugar was 268, even with the medications. The weight loss has taken time, but what has taken the most time is healing the long-term damage of diabetes and a poor diet .... I feel like I am in the bonus round of my life. I am walking the trails at our cabin, I am kayaking on the lake, I am down on the floor with my grandkids.*

Key Points

- The Mediterranean diet has been shown to reduce the risk of developing diabetes, lower HbA1c in people with type 2 diabetes, promote weight loss, and reduce the risk of major cardiovascular events. It has also been shown to increase telomere length, which is believed to be associated with a longer life expectancy.
- We encourage people with diabetes to seek the advice of a nutritionist for nutrition counseling. "Medical nutrition therapy" provides an opportunity for people with diabetes to be counselled about weight management, physical activity, caloric intake, and education about meal planning.
- If you need to lose weight, choose a diet that you will be able to adhere to long-term; make healthy choices including vitamins and minerals; eat your food slowly; and enjoy the ritual of sharing food with family or friends!

15

EXERCISE

It is better to discuss how far you have walked, than how little you have eaten.

—Elliott P. Joslin, MD

My kids have never seen me run. And I can now. And I love it.

—Corrine Tiliano, Participant in CDC's National Diabetes Prevention Program

The adoption of an exercise regimen is emphasized by clinicians as an important part of the treatment of people with diabetes. Exercise has a multitude of health benefits, including improvement in blood glucose control, weight maintenance, and a significant reduction in cardiovascular mortality. In addition, exercise often helps in dealing with depression.

A word about the **short-term** and **long-term** benefits of exercise in people with diabetes:

- With short-term exercise the muscles utilize more glucose. Even after one round of exercise, you will start to see a decrease in your glucose levels. Moreover, you will begin to feel your muscles strengthen and your mood improve. You will likely sleep better that night. But you may also have a few aches at first. Be patient, they are a sign you are making progress!
- Long-term, moderate-intensity, regular aerobic exercise has positive effects on muscle function that will lead to more efficient use of energy. In addition to lowering blood sugar, there is also a lowering of blood lipid concentrations, blood pressure and anxiety.

Both resistance training **and** aerobic exercise are recommended for optimal results

> Both resistance training and aerobic exercise are recommended for optimal results and weight loss.

and weight loss. In a study by Sigal and colleagues published in the *Annals of Internal Medicine* in 2007, it was noted that both aerobic and resistance training alone improved glycemic control in people with type 2 diabetes, but the improvements were greatest when individuals combined both aerobic and resistance exercises.

Long-term exercise not only lowers the levels of total cholesterol, "bad" LDL cholesterol and triglycerides, it also raises "good" HDL. It improves all aspects of your "lipid profile"!

Recommendations: Exercise

Before initiating an exercise regimen, it is strongly recommended that people with diabetes undergo a thorough history and physical examination and a resting electrocardiogram (EKG). Exercise stress testing is not routinely performed, but it is recommended if clinical features suggest someone has a higher risk of underlying coronary artery disease.

1. **Initial regimen**: A good initial regimen to implement is a 10-minute stretching and warm-up routine followed by 20 minutes of gentle exercise, such as walking or cycling, three to five times a week. People can then graduate to doing more strenuous activities.
2. **Routine**: The American Heart Association, American Diabetes Association and the American College of Sports Medicine recommend at least 150 minutes per week of moderately intense aerobic activity, ideally distributed over at least three days a week.
3. **Hydration**: It is important to be adequately hydrated before, during and after exercise.
4. **Glucose monitoring**: Monitoring blood glucose levels before, during and after exercise is important, especially in people who are taking insulin or sulfonylureas. This will inform the person of likely similar changes in blood sugar during subsequent exercise sessions. One can then incorporate dietary changes to prevent hypoglycemia. Ideally, prior to exercising, the blood glucose level should be in the 100 to 200 mg/dL range [5.5 to 11.0 mmol/L].
5. Both resistance training and aerobic **exercise** are recommended for optimal results in glycemic control and weight loss.

Resistance training does not require barbells or membership at a gym. Resistance bands can provide most adults with an adequate challenge.

We recommend that you talk with a trainer or physical therapist on how to add resistance training to your routine. One of the advantages of resistance bands is that you can take them when you travel and, for example, use them in your hotel room!

High-Intensity Interval Training

Although aerobic exercise is recommended for 30 minutes at least five days a week, High-Intensity Interval Training (HIIT, also called "Tabata") is an alternative for those who are pressed for time. It is an intense exercise approach that can provide the same benefit as 20 minutes of moderate exercise.

HIIT can be done, for example, on an exercise bike, jogging in place, calisthenics, using a jump-rope or running up and down stairs. An example of this is using a stationary bicycle, cycling for 30 seconds as intensely as possible using high resistance, followed by several minutes of slow cycling with low resistance for a few minutes. This sequence is then repeated. Repeating this eight times, for example, gives the individual an excellent aerobic workout. When done consistently for two weeks, it induces anerobic metabolism and becomes a true "fat-burning" exercise!

Sitting to Death

Prolonged sitting has been dubbed the "new smoking." There is strong evidence that prolonged sitting is associated with an increased risk of type 2 diabetes, cardiovascular disease, cancer and increased mortality. This risk is present even amongst people who exercise regularly. These findings culled from a meta-analysis were published in the *Annals of Internal Medicine* in 2015. The authors noted, however, that the association between sedentary behavior and all-cause mortality was greatest amongst people who exercised the least.

In a study published in 2020 in the *Journal of Gerontology*, the authors found that standing for 90 minutes per day reduced mortality by 37% and that even standing for as little as 30 minutes per day showed some reduction in mortality.

Patient Stories: The Power of Exercise

We share with you the story of a person with type 1 diabetes who not only embraces exercise but who has made exercise her "hobby" and has participated in many amateur races over the years.

LJ is now 53 years old and was diagnosed with type 1 diabetes 25 years ago, in 1995 when she presented with the classic symptoms of diabetes and a glucose of over 700 mg/dL. She has been taking a long-acting basal insulin and rapid-acting insulin at meals ever since and has maintained excellent control of her diabetes for the entire time. Her HbA1c levels have ranged between 5.9 and 7.4% for the past 25 years, with most being less than 6.8%. She has no microvascular complications of diabetes (retinopathy, nephropathy or neuropathy). She works full time as an industrial designer.

LJ was always active – she lifted weights and took step aerobics classes at a local gym, and had, in her "younger days," participated team sports. But things changed soon after she met her boyfriend in 2002. He too had been active in his younger days. He, his brother and a friend decided to start a triathlon team and they began training. LJ initially stood on the sidelines, only watching, but a year later, after being encouraged repeatedly by her boyfriend, she joined the team and participated in her first training triathlon, which comprised a half-mile swim, a 6-mile bike ride and a 3-mile run. After that, she said, "I caught the bug!"

Since 2003, she has participated in at least 50 triathlon races, and, more recently taken up cyclocross, too. Cyclocross is a cross between road racing and mountain biking, where competitors race laps around a course featuring a variety of surfaces – pavement, grass, sand, gravel, dirt – and during the race, they also must overcome some obstacles that may necessitate getting off and back on their bikes. She has now participated in about 70 of these races.

Today, there are sixty-two people on their team – some race triathlons, some do marathons, and some are cyclists only. In 2013, LJ fell off her bike while training to do a fundraising bike ride for the American Diabetes Association. She hurt her shoulder and then later developed a "frozen shoulder" (see page 98). She was devastated, but this did not set her back for long. While she had to temporarily stop racing, she continued to do whatever exercise she could, persisted with physical therapy and finally, three years later, she was fully recovered.

Now she is back racing and recently said to me, "This exercise and commitment to exercise has made a profound effect on my glucose control and my ability to maintain my sugars in good range almost all the time. And I need less insulin because of the exercise." She has won some medals too along the way. She recently participated in a 62 km cyclocross race. She told me, "Ten women started the race, and 3 finished. I was one of them and got the bronze medal for my efforts!"

More recently, she rode for seven hours to finish a 43-mile gravel ride in Vermont where 1500 people pre-registered. About 1200 competitors showed up to the snowy start line and only 838 riders finished in the grueling cold. She won the "lanterne rouge" for finishing last place with an Olympic cyclist running beside her cheering her on as she pedaled to the finish line. "It was an epic adventure where my diabetes management was the easy part!", she said afterwards!

When we met recently, she reminded me (MA) what I had said to her three days after she had been diagnosed with type 1 diabetes. "You told me," she said, "I don't want you to live your life any differently than any other 28-year-old. It might take a little more work, but you can do anything you put your mind to." She continued, "It's the words I've lived by since 1995 and I count myself lucky for having had you speak them to me, because they made (and still make) a difference every day."

Patient Stories: Olympic Gold

There are many competitive athletes who have type 1 diabetes and who achieve national and international recognition for their achievements. I was at a meeting discussing advances in diabetes a few years ago when the last speaker of the day went up to the podium. As soon as he was introduced, I knew that his story would not only be inspirational but would be a story I could recount to my patients to encourage them to "reach for the stars."

Gary Hall is a renowned Olympic swimmer who has represented the United States at none less than three Olympics. He comes from a family of Olympic swimmers – his father, grandfather and uncle all competed on the US Olympic Team. Gary represented the United States at the 1996 Olympics and won two silver medals.

In 1999, while training for the 2000 Olympics, Gary was diagnosed with type 1 diabetes. He was told initially by doctors that his swimming days were over and that he should not expect to swim competitively ever again. He was devastated. However, he did not accept that as an answer and sought a second opinion. He wound up seeing a colleague of mine who told him otherwise. With regular blood glucose testing (there was no CGM at the time) and multiple shots of insulin daily he restarted training. He worked up to training eight hours a day, getting out of the water to test his glucose every 45 minutes.

In 2000, he was not only back on the team representing the USA at the Olympics, but he also won a gold medal in the individual 50m freestyle, tying with his fellow US teammate Anthony Ervin. He won gold and silver in the team relays and a bronze medal in the individual 100 mg freestyle. And in 2004 he won gold again in the 50m freestyle, breaking his own record!

By the time he retired from competitive swimming in 2008 Gary, had won 10 Olympic medals, including five gold.

Take-Home Messages

- Anyone with diabetes who wants to exercise, can do so, and there is no limit to what they can do.
- People with diabetes can exercise competitively and, indeed, do so professionally too.
- Diabetes should not stop you from doing what you are passionate about and reaching for the stars.
- These individuals, and so many others, teach us that adversity is a gift – if we change the way we handle it – by treating it not as an obstacle but as a precious opportunity.

Key Points

- Exercise can be adopted by most people with type 1 and type 2 diabetes. Overall, it leads to better blood sugar control and lowers the risk of cardiovascular disease and death.
- Exercise also improves muscle tone, reduces stress and depression, lowers the risk of Alzheimer's Dementia, and contributes to an overall improvement in the quality of life and a boost in self-esteem.
- Your physician can help if you have health barriers to exercise. For example, for people with severe arthritis, there are forms of exercise that can be undertaken without causing and pain or discomfort, such as swimming or water aerobics. Upper body exercises can also be implemented.
- Many physicians use motivational interviewing to encourage regular exercise (see page 119). Your clinician may utilize this strategy to motivate you to exercise regularly.
- A helpful strategy is to consider one exercise you can do on a regular basis. If the answer is, "well, I could walk four days a week, 30 minutes each time," the clinician writes a prescription saying, "walk four times a week for 30 minutes each time." Number of refills – infinite!
- For many, having an exercise buddy is very useful. You can exercise together, or even connect remotely, to challenge one another to exercise at the same time or at different times and keep a tab on each other's success.
- Resistance training does not need barbells and membership at a gym. Resistance bands can provide most adults with an adequate challenge. We recommend that you talk with a trainer or physical therapist on how to add resistance training to your routine. One of the advantages of resistance bands is that you can take them when you travel and use them in your hotel room!
- Prolonged sitting has been dubbed as the "new smoking." There is strong evidence that prolonged sitting is associated with an increased risk of type 2 diabetes, cardiovascular disease, cancer and increased mortality. This risk is present even amongst people who exercise regularly.

16

INSULIN AND GLUCOSE CONTROL

I look upon the diabetic as a charioteer and his chariot as drawn by three steeds named (1) diet, (2) insulin and (3) exercise. It takes skill to drive one horse, intelligence to manage a team of two, but a man must be a very good teamster who can get all three to pull together and to succeed he needs instruction and practice.

—Elliot P. Joslin, MD

Insulin belongs to the world, not to me.

—Sir Frederick Grant Banting

Insulin was discovered in 1921 and became available for clinical use a year later. Leonard Thompson was the first person to be injected with insulin (see page 11). He was 14 at the time and lived for another 13 years before dying of pneumonia. Without insulin treatment, he likely would have only lived another six months after being diagnosed with type 1 diabetes!

The initial preparations - called "regular" or "soluble" insulin -were derived from animals and needed to be given multiple times a day as they were relatively short-acting. For the next 10 to 15 years, this type of insulin was the only product available for people with diabetes.

In the 1930s, efforts to produce a longer-acting insulin proved successful - this was achieved by mixing the insulin with protamine, resulting in an effect for up to 24 hours. It was felt that reducing the number of injections per day would not only be more convenient for people with diabetes but would also improve outcomes and quality of life. In addition, this insulin could be mixed with regular (short-acting) insulin in a single syringe.

We now know that minimizing the number of insulin injections for people who need full insulin replacement therapy, i.e. people with type 1 diabetes and some people with type 2 diabetes (notably those who have had type 2 diabetes for many years), is not appropriate, as this does not mimic the normal physiological release of insulin. Instead, multiple shots of insulin consisting of both long-acting and short-acting preparations are required to replicate normal physiology. To understand why, we need to think about how the pancreas normally produces insulin.

Normal Insulin Physiology

The function of insulin is to regulate the level of glucose – the main energy source for all cells – in the blood, by stimulating cells to take in glucose from the blood and use it to produce energy inside the cell. The normal pancreas secretes insulin in two ways; a constant "baseline" amount, known as **basal insulin secretion**, and a reactive secretion in response to a meal, which leads to increased glucose levels in the blood, known as **prandial insulin secretion**.

Basal secretion ensures there is always a small amount of insulin in circulation, including between meals and overnight. This prevents the body having to "switch" to alternative energy pathways, namely that of breaking down fat to produce ketones (an alternative energy source), and of the liver having to start producing glucose from other chemicals (one of its many essential roles!). Both pathways are essential during periods of starvation, to make sure cells get the glucose they need and don't fail or die!

Prandial secretion occurs after food is ingested, and glucose levels begin to rise, stimulating a rapid increase in insulin secretion by pancreatic beta-cells. The insulin circulating in the blood then stimulates most cells of the body to take in the plentiful glucose, ensuring levels do not rise above a certain threshold. As concentrations of glucose in the blood fall back to the normal range, insulin secretion is then rapidly switched off by the pancreas, ensuring glucose levels do not fall too low. An elegant system!

Ideal Insulin Therapy

Thus, in a person whose pancreas is not producing insulin, the ideal therapy would need to provide both basal and prandial insulin to try to

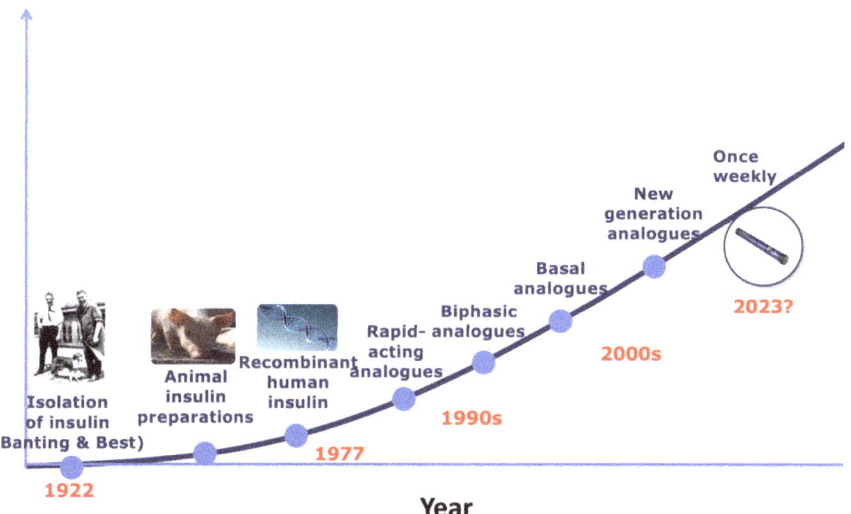

Reproduced and adapted with permission from Peter Kurtzhals, Novo Nordisk, Inc.

closely mimic normal physiology.

Of course, the insulin must be given by injection subcutaneously which is not the way insulin would normally be secreted (the normal pancreas secretes insulin directly into the blood stream). So, ideally, the insulin we inject should either start acting very quickly, to cover meals and then stop working once the food has been absorbed, or it needs to have a prolonged action that lasts 24 hours to mimic basal insulin secretion. This would ensure that glucose levels remain in a relatively normal range, or as close to normal as possible.

> *Insulin is not a cure for diabetes; it is a treatment. It enables the diabetic to burn sufficient carbohydrates so that proteins and fats may be added to the diet in sufficient quantities to provide energy for the economic burdens of life.*
> —Sir Frederick Grant Banting.

We have made incredible advances over the years in the development of these ideal insulins. One of the first major advances occurred in 1978 when scientists used technology called recombinant DNA to produce insulin that was identical to human insulin. They then added protamine or zinc to the insulin to extend its duration of action. These insulins became available for widespread use in 1982 and are still available and used today.

Insulin Analogs

Subsequently, however, scientists discovered that by replacing certain amino acids in the human insulin molecule they could alter the "pharmacokinetics" of the insulin to produce rapid-acting insulins as well as longer-acting basal insulins. Pharmacokinetics ("drug movements") describes the movement and action of drugs in the body; how rapidly or slowly is absorbed, gets into the blood stream, exerts its effects, is metabolized (broken down, usually to an inactive product) and finally, eliminated from the body.

These newer insulins are called insulin analogs and have become incorporated into the standard of clinical care in most countries of the world. There are rapid-acting analogs and long-acting (basal insulin) analogs which we use today.

Rapid-acting Insulin Analogs

These are rapidly absorbed after subcutaneous injection and start exerting an effect on glucose within 15 to 30 minutes after injection. They have their maximal effect within one to two hours after injection and are metabolized and eliminated within four hours. These insulins cover meals and are injected just before eating or even sometimes during the meal.

While not being quite as physiological as the "endogenous" insulin secreted by the normal pancreas, they are much more so in their

Comparison of Human Insulin and Insulin Analogs

Type	Onset of action	Peak action	Duration of action
Human regular	30–60 minutes	2–4 hours	8–10 hours
Human NPH*	1–2 hours	4–8 hours	10–20 hours
Rapid-acting analogs	5–15 minutes	1–2 hours	4–5 hours
Basal analogs**	1–2 hours	No peak	24+ hours

* Human NPH (Neutral Protamine Hagedorn) is the insulin bound to protamine. ** Refers to so-called 2nd generation basal insulin analogs.

kinetics than the original animal or human insulins.

Long-acting Insulin Analogs

These insulin analogs have a duration of action of more than 24 hours and are injected once a day. Their prolonged action is achieved either by delaying the absorption into the blood after injection, or by designing the insulin so that, after injection, it binds to albumin, the most abundant protein in the blood, preventing it exerting its effect until it is "released" by the albumin.

Long-acting insulin analogs are somewhat safer than rapid-acting analogs as their pharmacokinetics means they are less likely to cause hypoglycemia, one of the most serious and undesirable side effects of insulin treatment.

You can see from this table that human regular insulin, which is also given before meals, starts working much more slowly than the rapid-acting analog, has its peak effect much later and exerts its effects for much longer than the rapid-acting analogs. This is far less like normal endogenous insulin production in response to a meal than the modern rapid-acting analogs.

Similarly, the basal insulin analog's kinetics are much more like the normal basal production of insulin by the pancreatic beta cells.

New Types of Insulin

More recently, rapid-acting insulin analogs have been modified to start working even more quickly after injection - these formulations are available today for clinical use. Scientists at Stanford University, however, are working on the development of an **ultrafast** acting insulin whose onset of action is four times faster than the currently available rapid-acting insulin analogs. They screened many compounds and found one which, when added to the insulin, allows the insulin to act "ultra-" rapidly after injection. This has been shown to be highly effective in pigs and holds promise for use in humans in the near future.

Another advance in insulin therapy is the development of a long-acting basal insulin that can be given once a week instead of once a day. This is currently being studied in human trials and the preliminary findings are encouraging and have demonstrated that this insulin is as safe as basal insulins given once a day.

Does Insulin Have to be Injected?

As injection is a concern for many people, this has been the subject of intense research for many years and continues to keep scientists up at night.

There is an **inhaled form of insulin** which has been approved for clinical use by the US Food and Drug Administration (FDA). This is a very rapid-acting insulin and is given with meals. This insulin is breathed into the lungs with an inhaler much like inhalers used for asthma. Once in the lungs, the insulin is absorbed into the bloodstream. This insulin can be used instead of rapid-acting insulin analogs given by injection, but if one needs a long-acting insulin, that still requires injection. Inhaled insulin is contraindicated in people who smoke, or who have lung problems like asthma, chronic bronchitis, or chronic obstructive pulmonary disease (COPD). It is not used very extensively in the US. Prior to using it, it is necessary to have lung function tests, which should be repeated periodically while inhaled insulin is being used.

At present insulin cannot be taken by mouth. If given orally, it is degraded by the acid in the stomach before it can be absorbed to exert its effect. However, scientists are working on an oral insulin preparation that is coated with a protective substance that allows it to survive the acidic stomach so it can then be absorbed in the small intestine.

Scientists are working on an oral insulin preparation that is coated with a protective substance to prevent it being broken down by stomach acid, then allowing it to be absorbed in the small intestine.

Insulin Delivery

As stated above, people with type 1 diabetes need insulin to be given in a way that is as close to natural physiology as possible. This means with each meal and usually also one long-acting injection per day. To make things more convenient, these insulins can be administered using **pen devices** which are much easier to use then vials and syringes. The needles on the pens are so thin and short so as to make the injection almost painless.

Another way in which this insulin is delivered is via an **insulin infusion pump**. These pumps continuously deliver insulin throughout the day and night and can also be used to give a "bolus" or prandial doses when meals are eaten. Only short-acting or rapid-acting insulin is used in these pumps. Most people who use pumps have type 1 diabetes, but some people with type 2 diabetes that require multiple shots of insulin also take advantage of this method of insulin delivery.

Insulin in Type 2 Diabetes

When people with type 2 diabetes cannot achieve their glucose goals with two or three medications, it is usually time to add insulin to their treatment regimen. In most cases, they may only require basal insulin, which would then be added to the other medications they are taking (see page 151). It is not uncommon for people who are taking medications like metformin, GLP-1 receptor agonists, and SGLT-2 inhibitors, to require additional basal insulin treatment to help them achieve their target glucose levels. Basal insulin is usually taken at night before going to bed.

There are injectable preparations that contain both basal insulin and GLP-1 receptor agonists. These "fixed ratio" products enable injection of two medications at once and are very effective at lowering glucose levels in the appropriate circumstances in people with type 2 diabetes.

Hypoglycemia

One of the common side effects of insulin treatment is low blood glucose, or hypoglycemia. We categorize the severity as follows in people with diabetes:

1. **Mild** (level 1) hypoglycemia: glucose levels below 70 mg/dL or 3.9 mmol/L.
2. **Serious** (level 2) hypoglycemia: glucose levels below 54 mg/dL or 3.0 mmol/L.
3. **Severe** (level 3) hypoglycemia: when the individual is not able to self-treat the hypoglycemia and requires help from another person or emergency room treatment.

Usually, people with glucose levels in these ranges can treat themselves. A hypoglycemic event in which the individual is unable to treat themselves is considered severe hypoglycemia. If untreated it can lead to a hypoglycemic coma.

Symptoms

The most common symptoms include increasing perspiration, sensation of a more rapid heartbeat (palpitations), increasing anxiety and shakiness. People with diabetes - and often their family members - realize that these symptoms mean they need to ingest glucose to bring their blood glucose levels up.

If glucose levels drop to a dangerous level, people develop cognitive dysfunction, an inability to think clearly, and sometimes even behave inappropriately, for example they become more aggressive or say inappropriate things. These symptoms are serious and are usually a sign of severe hypoglycemia.

> People with long-standing diabetes may lose the early "classic" symptoms of hypoglycemia – referred to as "hypoglycemic unawareness." In such people, the first symptom of hypoglycemia may be cognitive dysfunction.

Treatment

The most effective treatment for hypoglycemia includes orange juice, milk, and sugary beverages like Coca-Cola. We usually recommend "**the rule of 15**" for treating the symptoms:

1. Take 15 grams of glucose;
2. Wait 15 minutes;
3. Recheck your blood glucose levels and if they are not above 70 mg/dL or 3.9 mmol/L, take another 15 grams.

Over time, people with long-standing diabetes or those who have frequent episodes of hypoglycemia may lose the typical symptoms of hypoglycemia described above, and cognitive dysfunction may be the first clinical manifestation of low glucose levels. This is dangerous, as the "warning signs" have been lost. Unless people are aware of this, they may not necessarily treat the hypoglycemic episodes themselves. This can of course lead to severe hypoglycemia, culminating in coma or convulsions. In these situations, the individual needs help - either from a friend, partner or EMT (emergency medical team) or sometimes intravenous glucose treatment in an emergency room.

Prevention

Your clinician (primary care physician, nurse practitioner, physician assistant, diabetologist or diabetes educator) will undoubtedly go over the right way to administer insulin in relation to food and exercise and ensure that there is a reduced chance of experiencing hypoglycemia. Using insulin analogs and taking insulin in a way that mimics the production of insulin by the pancreas greatly reduces the risk of hypoglycemia.

People taking insulin are often prescribed **glucagon**, a hormone that does the opposite of what insulin does; it raises blood glucose levels. This is usually given to a person who is not able to self-treat the episode of hypoglycemia by a partner or friend. For many years glucagon had to be given by injection but recently a nasal form of glucagon was approved by the FDA for clinical use.

Insulin Therapy and Weight Gain

Unfortunately, weight gain of approximately 3 to 5 pounds [1.4–2.3 kg] is a common side effect of insulin therapy. With insulin treatment, glucose can enter the cells and blood glucose levels drop – this is the intention of treatment. If, however, one consumes more calories than the body needs, the glucose that the cells don't use accumulates as fat which leads to weight gain.

To minimize weight gain we recommend that you watch your caloric intake more carefully and maintain an active lifestyle.

Monitoring Blood Glucose

For many years the only way people could check their glucose levels was to measure the amount of glucose in their urine (when glucose levels in the blood exceed a certain level, it "spills over" through the kidney and into the urine).

In the 1920s and 1930s this had to be done by putting the urine in a test tube, adding a specific reagent to it, boiling up the urine and looking at the color that it changed to. In the 1960s, this was replaced by small absorbent strips that contained a reagent that reacts with glucose and changes color, roughly proportional to the amount of glucose present.

In the 1970s, **fingerstick glucose monitoring** was introduced and represented a major advance in the ability to monitor glucose levels. For the first time, people with diabetes could measure the glucose level quantitatively. Fingerstick glucose technology has advanced rapidly as have the meters used to measure glucose levels. Using current devices, a tiny drop of blood – less than 15 microliters (uL) – on a strip that connects to a meter can provide an accurate measurement of the glucose reading within seconds of the test being done.

Glucose Monitoring Devices

Even further advances in glucose measurement technology are now available for widespread use. These are referred to as to **continuous glucose monitoring** (CGM) devices or **flash glucose monitoring** (FGM) devices.

Today, we no longer need to do a fingerstick to measure glucose levels. We can wear a device called a glucose sensor, which remains attached to the body for up to two weeks at a time and which provides a continuous measurement of glucose readings. These sensors are easy to insert and provide very accurate readings of glucose. They can be connected via Bluetooth to smart phones or even smart watches and provide continuous information about glucose levels in the blood. Some sensors can be embedded under the skin with a small incision and are then replaced every three months.

Over the last few years researchers have been able to "connect" these CGM devices with insulin pumps and, using software technology, enable the pumps to increase or decrease basal insulin secretion based on the glucose levels received from the CGM device. This is what we call "closing the loop." Technology is advancing at a rapid pace, and soon we hope to see the **artificial pancreas** available for clinical use. This will automate not only basal secretion of insulin by the pump but also prandial secretion of insulin which will cover meals, and which will result in almost totally normal glucose levels with no hypoglycemia or hyperglycemia!

Hemoglobin A1c (HbA1c)

In the 1970s, a test for hemoglobin HbA1c was introduced. This is a test for glucose bound to hemoglobin (the oxygen-carrying protein in red blood cells) that reflects the average glucose control over the preceding few months. Since its discovery, it has been the gold standard test used in both clinical care and in research.

Because glucose bonds irreversibly to hemoglobin, HbA1c lasts as long as the red cells lifespan of up to 120 days. Measuring a component of glucose on hemoglobin provides an estimate of overall glucose control during this period. This test is used together with glucose monitoring to assess how well controlled your diabetes is.

The Goals of Glucose Control

Now that we can accurately measure glucose levels in the blood and do tests like HbA1c to measure long-term glucose control, we need to understand what our goals of treatment should be. Most international organizations believe that every individual should achieve the best possible glucose control that she or he can achieve providing this can be done safely, in other words without causing an unacceptable risk of hypoglycemia.

> Most organizations believe that everyone should achieve the best possible glucose control that she or he can, whilst being careful to avoid the risk of hypoglycemia.

For most people, the goal is a HbA1c of less than 7%. In addition, glucose levels on waking and before meals should be between 80 and 130 mg/dL [4.4–7.2 mmol/L], and two hours after meals less than 180 mg/dL [10.0 mmol/L]. This is the recommendation of the American Diabetes Association and is shared by many other organizations around the world. Some organizations, like the American Association of Clinical Endocrinologists, believe an ideal HbA1c should be 6.5% or less, but, once again, with the caveat that this should be achieved safely, avoiding hypoglycemia.

With the advent of CGM we are now looking at another way to assess glucose control. This is called "**time in range**" and refers to what percentage of time blood glucose levels are in an acceptable range, i.e., between 70 and 180 mg/dL [3.9–10.0 mmol/L] or above or below that range. Ideally, one should have glucose levels in range approximately 70% of the time (more than this if the individual is pregnant). Seeing this information allows the consultant to provide advice to the patient regarding changes in both insulin dose and food intake. It also provides the user with important feedback to improve their glucose control.

Individualized Goals

All diabetes-related organizations also believe that we need to individualize treatment goals. For some people, **tight glucose control**, as outlined above should be aggressively pursued. This applies to younger individuals, people who have no other illnesses or complications of diabetes, and who are expected to live a normal life span despite their diabetes.

However, these goals may not be appropriate for others, including elderly people, or people who have unfortunately developed many complications of diabetes or may have other illnesses that are associated with a shorter life expectancy. Other people who may not be candidates for very tight glucose control include people who have experienced recurrent episodes of severe hypoglycemia.

It is important that you talk to your doctor about glucose control and what your targets should be. You can then do your best to achieve the best possible glucose without putting yourself at increased risk for other complications like hypoglycemia.

Why is Good Glucose Control So Important?

Prior to the discovery of insulin, people who developed type 1 diabetes had a life expectancy of roughly six months after diagnosis! The only treatment available was a very low-carbohydrate or ketogenic diet, essentially a starvation diet.

> We now have excellent evidence that good glucose control reduces the risk for the development and progression of both microvascular and macrovascular complications.

Once insulin became available, death from the acute complications of diabetes could be avoided, and people survived for many years. However, it was then noticed that people with diabetes were developing other complications, so-called microvascular complications, where diabetes affects the small blood vessels of the body, particularly the eye, kidney and peripheral nerves of the limbs. People with diabetes were developing blindness, end-stage kidney disease, and diminished sensation in the feet at increased rates. They were also developing large vessel (macrovascular) disease, including cardiovascular and peripheral vascular disease, at higher rates than the normal population.

Clinicians taking care of people with diabetes then began to ask the question, "could good glucose control improve outcomes and reduce the risk for the development or progression of these complications?" With better insulins available, the ability for people to monitor their blood glucoses accurately and the HbA1c test that measured long-term glucose control, the question could potentially be answered. So, in the 1970s and 80s, studies were started to answer these questions.

In the early 1990s, the first well-controlled study to address this was published. It was called the Diabetes Control and Complications Trial (DCCT), and it compared tight glucose control with the conventional and less tight control in people with type 1 diabetes. And It showed unequivocally that tight glucose control significantly reduced the risk for the development and progression of the microvascular complications of diabetes. A similar study in people with type 2 diabetes was published a few years later with the same results. This was the United Kingdom Prospective Diabetes Study (UKPDS).

So, we now have excellent evidence that good glucose control reduces the risk for the development and progression of both microvascular and macrovascular complications. It therefore goes without saying that *anyone who develops diabetes should strive to achieve the best possible control they can.*

Even If you have had diabetes for many years and have struggled with, or are struggling with, controlling your blood glucose, improving your glucose control still reduces the risk for the development or progression of microvascular complications. Improving glucose control may not affect the risk for cardiovascular disease but remember that there are also other medications used to reduce risk for cardiovascular disease.

These include statins to lower cholesterol and good blood pressure lowering drugs. Smoking remains a significant risk factor for the development of cardiovascular disease and peripheral vascular disease and avoidance of smoking and cessation of smoking is to bc encouraged. In fact, a

An important study from Denmark called the Steno 2 study published in the *New England Journal of Medicine* in 2008 showed that aggressive management of all cardiovascular risk factors, including glucose, cholesterol, blood pressure and smoking cessation, reduced the risk for a cardiovascular event and mortality by a staggering 50%!

study from Denmark called the Steno 2 study published in the *New England Journal of Medicine* in 2008 showed that aggressive management of all cardiovascular risk factors, including glucose, cholesterol, blood pressure and smoking cessation, reduced the risk for a cardiovascular event and mortality by a staggering 50%!

Patient Stories: Starting Insulin

The first patient is EI, a 56-year-old African American male nurse who was diagnosed with type 2 diabetes eight years ago. At the time of diagnosis, he had no symptoms – the diagnosis was made by routine blood tests. His HbA1c at diagnosis was 7.9%. Rather than start medications immediately, he elected to follow a reduced carbohydrate diet and started a regular exercise program that included both aerobic and resistance training. He lost 10 pounds [4.5 kg] and his HbA1c came down to 7.3%. In consultation with his primary care physician, he agreed to start metformin and three months later his HbA1c was 6.8%. His diabetes remained stable for the next three years.

At a routine follow-up appointment at that time his HbA1c had increased to 7.5% even though he had continued to take metformin and followed his diet and exercise program diligently. He had no complications related to diabetes. Once again, in consultation with his physician he elected to add a GLP-1 receptor agonist to his treatment regimen. He tolerated this medication well and lost another 10 pounds. His HbA1c dropped to 6.7%.

Three months prior to his visit with one of us he was seen for a follow-up visit and commented that he was a little more thirsty than usual and that he had noted that his blood glucose readings in the morning on waking had increased gradually over the preceding six months from the low 120s to the 170s. He had not gained any weight, was still exercising, and trying to limit his carbohydrate intake. His primary care physician thought he should start basal insulin to lower the fasting glucose readings and referred him for a second opinion. His HbA1c had risen to 7.8%.

When one of us met him, he felt frustrated that his morning glucoses had risen, even though he had not changed any aspects of his self-care or medications. His weight was steady at 202 pounds [91.6 kg] and his height 5’8” giving him a BMI of 30.4 kg/m^2.

I informed him that unfortunately this is the natural history of the disease. In other words, with the passage of time, type 2 diabetes progresses and approximately 50% of people will require insulin being added to their treatment regimen (this was demonstrated in the landmark trial called the United Kingdom Prospective Diabetes Study (UKPDS; see page 143). The elevated fasting glucose is caused by the liver producing excess glucose overnight, a very common scenario.

He was somewhat disappointed but said "Doctor, you are the expert, and I'll listen to your advice. But is this injection painful? Who will teach me to do it correctly? Are there the side effects?"

We discussed all of this in detail with him and he was referred to the diabetes nurse educator who went over all aspects of the administration of insulin with a pen device, and potential side effects of treatment, in particular hypoglycemia. He was also advised that we start the insulin at a low dose to avoid any risk of hypoglycemia and titrate the dose up gradually to achieve the target fasting glucose goal, which is usually between 80 and 130 mg/dL.

He was started on a small dose of a basal insulin analog (ten units) and taught how to increase the dose in small increments (two units) every two to four days to achieve his target glucose level. One month later he was taking 20 units and his morning glucose levels were down to 140 mg/dL. Two months later he walked into the office with a smile on his face and said "Doc, we did it! Taking insulin is really no big deal. I have had no side effects of treatment. I am now taking 26 units and my morning sugars are around 120 mg/dL!" His repeat HbA1c was now 6.9%, down from 7.8% prior to the start of insulin.

Take-Home Messages

- Type 2 diabetes is a progressive disease and additional treatments, including insulin, are often required.
- Although people are often reluctant to start insulin, once they do so, they tolerate it exceedingly well and are very satisfied to see the therapeutic benefit.
- Injecting insulin with the new pen devices and very thin needles is less painful than doing fingerstick pricking to measure the blood glucose.
- If insulin is needed, it is better to start sooner than later and not partake in what is referred to as "clinical inertia" on the part of both patient and clinician.

Patient Stories: Coming Off Insulin

AK is an 85-year-old woman of Asian American descent. She has had type 2 diabetes for 25 years. She has also had cardiovascular disease for many years, which manifested as an episode of chest pain diagnosed as unstable angina. This led to an emergency cardiac catheterization at which time three stents were deployed in her coronary arteries. Since that time, she has had no chest pain.

She takes medications for high blood pressure and elevated cholesterol. With regard to diabetes-specific complications, she has peripheral neuropathy that does not bother her too much. She takes good care of her feet, sees a podiatrist regularly, has annual dilated eye examinations and has no visual symptoms or evidence of retinopathy.

When initially diagnosed with diabetes she was started on metformin. Three years later she needed to add another medication and five years later she started taking basal insulin. About ten years ago she required the addition of insulin at meals and her oral anti-diabetes medications were stopped. At present she takes 25 units of basal insulin at night and anywhere between four and eight units of rapid-acting insulin with each meal. She tests her glucose three to four times daily.

AK lives alone, does all her own housework and cooking, and manages all her activities of daily living. She goes for a walk every day with her dog. She is well-informed about carbohydrates, fats and proteins and the need to be as consistent as possible with her intake of carbohydrate at meals to best avoid hypoglycemia.

She was seen for a routine visit by one of us and arrived accompanied by her daughter, who had a worried look on her face. When asked how Mrs. AK was, her daughter started talking before her mother and stated, "Doctor, I am a little concerned. My mom has had a few "spells" lately – for example, when we were out shopping last week, she suddenly felt dizzy and lightheaded and had to have some orange juice, after which she felt better. She also reported that the other night she had woken in the middle of the night sweaty and shaky, and once again had taken some orange juice, and shortly after that, she felt better. I think she is having too many lows and I am worried."

AK confirmed the comments of her daughter and added, "Oh, doctor, this has been happening for a few months now. I kept a log of my sugars and I've brought it with me to show you. What do you think I should do?"

We took a look at her glucose logs (units are in mg/dL – divide by 18 to convert to mmol/L):

	Before breakfast	Before lunch	Before dinner	Before bed
Monday	85	129	130	150
Tuesday	99	110	99	145
Wednesday	76	65*	88	162
Thursday	108	132	129	154
Friday	115	86	130	167
Saturday	Forgot to test	Out shopping	72	129**
Sunday	92	62***	150	No test

* Felt a little lightheaded and had 4 oz of orange juice
** Woke during the night sweaty and shaky and had 4 oz orange juice.
*** Did not eat breakfast; did not take insulin at breakfast but had no symptoms at lunch.

What was interesting is that she had clearly had at least two documented hypoglycemic episodes (i.e., glucose under 70 mg/dL or 3.9 mmol/L) according to these logs, one of which had apparently occurred with no symptoms. This was on Sunday when she recorded a blood glucose level of 62 mg/dL [3.4 mmol/L], before eating lunch.

Overall, her glucose levels for someone of her age (85 years) and with underlying cardiovascular disease were too low, even potentially dangerously low!

Clinical examination that day revealed someone who looked well and who's blood pressure was excellent. She weighed 144 pounds [65.3 kg]; her height was 5'2", which gave her a BMI of 26 kg/m^2. Her physical examination was normal apart from findings consistent with peripheral neuropathy.

Her laboratory tests revealed a glucose level of 70 mg/dL [3.9 mmol/L] and a HbA1c of 6.4%. She had impaired kidney function tests but normal liver function tests.

The conversation that ensued was interesting. I told AK that her diabetes control was now too good! "What?!", she said, "after all these years of trying to maintain good glucose control you are telling me that my control is too good?" As I explained things, both she and her daughter began to understand. "Mrs. AK," I said, "there comes a time when rarely we have to advise people that very good control may be associated with an increased risk of hypoglycemia, which is what has happened to you. Part of the reason is that your kidneys are not working as well as they used to, and this has two effects. First, the insulin you inject is taking longer to be eliminated by the kidneys, meaning it is in the blood longer and has a longer effect of lowering glucose. Second, one of the functions of the kidneys is to produce a little glucose – what we call "gluconeogenesis," and as we age, they produce less. Another cause of lower glucose."

> *As a result of these factors, your glucose levels are going too low, causing hypoglycemia. In someone of your age with underlying cardiovascular disease, this is potentially more life-threatening in the short-term than having mildly elevated glucose.*

So, what was the solution? We decided there and then to radically change her treatment. The dose of the long-acting insulin was decreased from 25 units to 20 units. Additionally, we stopped all rapid-acting insulin and instead started her on a GLP-1 receptor agonist, which she injected once a week. She was willing to accept potential side effects of the new medication and understood that if she ate smaller meals and avoided excessive fatty food the chances of her developing nausea were significantly reduced. She was delighted that she would now be taking one injection per day instead of four injections a day. The additional weekly injection she said, with a smile, was "no big deal"!

She was seen one month later. There had been no episodes of hypoglycemia. Her lowest glucose recorded was 95 mg/dL [5.3 mmol/L] and her highest was 166 mg/dL [9.2 mmol/L]. Three months later, she announced that there had been no "spells" or further episodes of hypoglycemia. She was tolerating her medications well and continued to lead an active and normal life. We repeated her HbA1c which was now 7.2% – totally acceptable for someone of her age and duration of diabetes with cardiovascular disease.

Take-Home Messages

- As people age the goals for glucose control change, especially if there are other conditions present like cardiovascular disease. In these circumstances, higher glucose readings, if they are generally under 200 mg/dL [11.1 mmol/L], are acceptable.
- As kidney function deteriorates, there is often a need for less insulin because the insulin is metabolized more slowly, and the kidneys no longer contribute as much to glucose production.
- It is extremely important to avoid hypoglycemia in elderly people – glucose monitoring becomes even more important because often people with long-standing diabetes don't feel the typical symptoms of

a low glucose.

- In situations like this we are fortunate to now have alternatives to insulin that are much less likely to result in hypoglycemia. Another advantage of using a GLP-1 receptor agonist in this patient is that this class of medications is known to confer significant cardiovascular benefit, separate from their glucose-lowering effect. An excellent bonus!

Key Points

- Prior to the discovery of insulin, people who developed type 1 diabetes had a life expectancy of roughly six months - the only treatment was a very low-carbohydrate or ketogenic diet, essentially a starvation diet.
- Once insulin became available, death from the acute complications of diabetes could be avoided, and people survived for many years.
- The most effective treatment for hypoglycemia includes orange juice, milk, and sugary beverages like Coca-Cola. We usually recommend the "rule of 15" for treating the symptoms: take 15 grams of glucose, wait 15 minutes, recheck your blood glucose levels and if they are not above 70 mg/dL [3.9 mmol/L], take another 15 g of glucose.
- The Danish Steno 2 study published in the *New England Journal of Medicine* in 2008 showed that aggressive management of all cardiovascular risk factors, including glucose, cholesterol, blood pressure and smoking cessation, reduced the risk for a cardiovascular event and mortality by a staggering 50%!
- Even if you have struggled for many years with glucose control, and are still struggling, improving it will still reduce your risk for the development or progression of microvascular complications. It really is worth the effort!

17

NON-INSULIN MEDICATIONS

We cannot change the cards we are dealt, just how we play the hand.

—Randy Pausch

When diet and exercise have failed to control glucose levels, it is time to start medication. Fifty years ago, in the US, there were only two choices: insulin or sulfonylureas. Today, there are thankfully many more very effective classes of medications available for use.

'Older' Non-insulin Medications Used in Type 2 Diabetes

	Metformin	Thiazolidinediones	Sulphonylureas	Alpha-glucosidase inhibitors
Glucose-lowering efficacy	High	High	High	Moderate
Hypoglycemia	No	No	Yes	No
Effect on weight	Neutral mainly, occasionally some loss	Gain	Gain	Neutral
Possible side-effects	Diarrhea, flatulence	Fluid retention, bone fractures	Nausea	Diarrhea, flatulence

Adapted from the ASCEND (Academy for Science and Continuing Education in Diabetes and Obesity) Program. http://www.ASCEND-diabetes-obesity.com.

Metformin

The first-line medication for most people is metformin. It was first approved for use in other parts of the world in the 1950s but only became available in the US in the 1990s.

Interestingly, metformin was originally derived from the plant *Galega officinalis*, known as "goat's rue" or "French lilac." In the 18th century, this plant was used to treat the symptoms of diabetes, but it was very toxic and had many side effects. In the 1940s, the beneficial chemical of the plant was isolated and synthesized and subsequently developed as a medication to treat diabetes. It was originally called *glucophage* – "glucose eater!"

Mechanism

Metformin works by helping the insulin in the body work more effectively. The precise mechanism of action is still not completely understood after more than 60 years of clinical use, but in a recent publication in the journal *Diabetes Care* scientists reported that metformin increased the excretion of blood sugar from the large intestine into the stool. This is a new discovery and clearly needs to be validated.

Metformin has some other potential benefits beyond lowering blood sugar levels. For example, in a study published in the journal *Diabetes Care* in 2020, the authors of the "Sydney Memory and Ageing Study" reported that cognitive decline and development of dementia was lower in elderly people with diabetes who took metformin.

Metformin has also attracted the attention of scientists studying ageing. It may increase telomere length and favorably affect other cellular markers of ageing. We should expect more definitive answers as to whether it actually increases life expectancy in humans in the near future.

Intriguing preliminary research suggests that people who take metformin may also have a lower risk of developing certain malignancies including cancers of the breast, liver, colon, prostate and pancreas.

Side Effects

The major side effect of metformin is diarrhea – this can often be avoided if the drug is started at a low dose and the dose is increased slowly. There is also a long-acting form of metformin that has fewer side effects than the original medication. Metformin should not be used in people who have significantly impaired kidney function.

Additional Medications

If metformin alone is not adequate to control blood glucose levels (see page 141), there are a variety of other medications that can be added to it.

'Newer' Non-insulin Medications Used in Type 2 Diabetes

	DPP-4 inhibitors	GLP-1 receptor agonists	SGLT-2 inhibitors
Glucose-lowering Efficacy	Moderate	High	Moderate
Hypoglycemia	No	No	No
Effect on Weight	Neutral	Loss	Loss
Possible side-effects	Joint pain	Nausea, diarrhea or constipation	Genitourinary infections; loss of blood fluid volume

Adapted from the ASCEND (Academy for Science and Continuing Education in Diabetes and Obesity) Program. http://www.ASCEND-diabetes-obesity.com.

When considering which to use for a particular patient, we assess:

- the **effectiveness** of the drug;
- its **safety**, in particular the risk of hypoglycemia;
- **side effects**; and
- other potential **additional benefits** the medication offers, such as weight loss and cardiovascular benefit (remember that cardiovascular disease is at least two times more likely to occur in people whose diabetes is not well controlled).

Over the past 15 years we have seen new medications come to market that are safer to use, do not cause hypoglycemia (when used alone or with metformin), can cause weight loss, and have the added benefit of reducing the risk for cardiovascular disease. There are two classes of medications that have been shown to reduce the risk for cardiovascular disease: glucagon-like peptide-1 (GLP-1) receptor agonists and sodium-glucose cotransporter-2 (SGLT-2) inhibitors.

GLP-1 Receptor Agonists

The research leading to the discovery of GLP-1 began in the 1960s thanks to new technology allowing us to accurately measure the amount of insulin in the blood (see page 139). Scientists discovered that the amount of insulin produced by the pancreas was much greater if glucose was taken orally compared to being injected intravenously (into a vein). They called this the **incretin effect**. Further research into this led to the identification of GLP-1 and its chemical structure in the 1980s.

Mechanism

Subsequently, numerous and elegant studies done by a number of scientists all over the world revealed how the hormone works. These scientists, including Drs. Daniel Drucker, Joel Habener, Jens Juul Holst and Michael Nauck, have received many major awards for their seminal work. They discovered that GLP-1 is a hormone that is produced by cells in the intestine when food enters the stomach. This hormone not only stimulates insulin production from the pancreas, but has many other actions, including suppression of the production of another hormone, **glucagon**, also produced in the pancreas. Glucagon has anti-insulin effects, including:

- Decreased glucose production by the liver.
- Slowed emptying of the stomach so food enters the blood stream more slowly.
- Decreased appetite.

GLP-1 has a very short half-life and thus cannot be used for clinical purposes. It is rapidly degraded by an enzyme called dipeptidyl peptidase-4 (DPP-4). It was also discovered that production of GLP-1 is decreased in people with type 2 diabetes, thereby further reducing the amount of insulin produced by the pancreas in response to eating. So, what was needed for an effective drug was a similar protein to GLP-1 that mimics its actions by stimulating the same cell receptors - what we call a "receptor agonist" - but that is not so rapidly degraded by DPP-4.

> GLP-1 receptor agonists stimulate the optimal amount of insulin release such that they will not cause hypoglycemia when used alone or with metformin.

Gila Monster

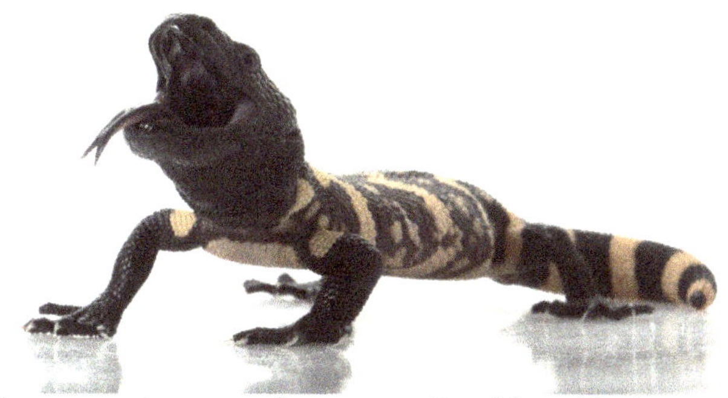

The Gila monster is a type of venomous lizard found in the Southwestern United States and northwestern Mexican state of Sonora.

Exenatide

A major step occurred in 1992 when Dr. John Eng, working at the Veterans Administration Medical Center in the Bronx, New York, isolated a substance from the saliva of a reptile called the **Gila monster**. It is a large venomous lizard native to the southwestern United States and northwestern Mexican state of Sonora. The saliva of this animal contains a hormone called **exendin-4**, which the Gila monster needs to digest its prey.

Dr. Eng discovered that this hormone stimulated insulin secretion from the pancreas of rats and had a variety of other effects, including blocking excessive glucose production by the liver, slowing the emptying of food from the stomach, and increasing satiety (sense of fullness after eating).

A synthetic form of this hormone – **exenatide** – was the first GLP-1 receptor agonist to become available for clinical use. There are now others, some that are given once a day, some only once a week. Recently, an oral form – as effective as the injectable form – has been approved for clinical use.

GLP-1 receptor agonists are a great step forward for diabetes management as they stimulate the optimal amount of insulin release such that they will not cause hypoglycemia when used alone or with metformin.

Side Effects

> A GLP-1 receptor agonist, dulaglutide, marketed as Trulicity in the USA, has recently been shown to decrease the risk of developing cognitive decline by 14% when compared to people who did not take this medication. This finding requires further validation.

GLP-1 receptor agonists, whether taken orally or by injection, may initially cause nausea and other gastrointestinal problems such as diarrhea or constipation. These side effects, however, can be minimized by starting the drug at a low dose and increasing it slowly and by eating smaller meals and consuming fewer fatty foods.

Contraindications

GLP-1 receptor agonists are contraindicated in people who have a history of pancreatitis, or if they have a very rare form of thyroid cancer called medullary carcinoma (or have a family history of this tumor), as there has been concern they can exacerbate or increase the risk of these conditions. In our experience, these drugs have not caused either of these and indeed long-term studies have confirmed their safety. However, we suggest that you discuss this with your clinician if you have any concerns.

SGLT-2 Inhibitors

The other class of medication shown to have a cardiovascular benefit are the SGLT-2 inhibitors. The first of these was approved for use by the Food and Drug Administration (FDA) in 2013. SGLT-2 inhibitors work by blocking the reabsorption of glucose from the kidneys, causing glucose to be excreted in the urine, thereby lowering blood glucose levels.

Sodium-glucose Transporter Proteins

The kidneys filter up to 150 quarts [170 liters] of blood every day, in order to filter out unwanted toxins into urine, prevent the loss of valuable substances and also to help keep blood volume (and therefore blood pressure) in balance.

In its elegant but complex filtration system, the kidney initially filters glucose out of the blood, and then reabsorbs it back into the blood as the urine is concentrated. After all, glucose is the body's prime source of energy! Loss of glucose in the urine (known as **glycosuria**) is a loss of high-energy fuel. However, enhancing glucose loss in the urine is a possible way to lower blood glucose in people with diabetes and elevated blood glucose levels.

For many years, the exact mechanism of glucose reabsorption was not understood. In the 1980s, however, researchers discovered a key protein involved: the sodium-glucose transporter protein (SGLT). They also discovered two types, one found mainly in the intestine (type 1) and the other found mainly in the kidneys (type 2).

Origin and Mechanism

Phlorizin is a natural product found in the bark of pear, apple, cherry and other fruit trees. It was first isolated from the bark of the apple tree in 1835. When given to animals, it led to increased glycosuria and weight loss. It was first tested in humans in the 1930s.

After the discovery of sodium-glucose transporter proteins, it was discovered that phlorizin blocked these proteins, thereby preventing the kidney's reabsorption of glucose from the urine back into the blood. However, phlorizin is not an effective drug because it is poorly absorbed from the gut in humans and affects glucose reabsorption from other organs apart from the kidney.

The SGLT-2 inhibitors are safer derivatives of phlorizin that specifically act in the kidney. People taking these medications for diabetes can lose up to 50 grams of glucose a day in their urine!

Side Effects

Like GLP-1 receptor agonists, SGLT-2 inhibitors also do not cause hypoglycemia when used alone or with GLP-1 receptor agonists or with metformin. They also cause weight loss, and more recently have been shown to be of benefit to people who have congestive heart failure or people with chronic kidney disease. They are associated with a slight increased risk of urinary tract and genital infections, but the risk is low and can be reduced with simple hygienic measures.

Other Medications

Other medications used to lower glucose levels in people with type 2 diabetes include dipeptidyl peptidase-4 (DPP-4) inhibitors, sulfonylureas, thiazolidinediones, alpha-glucosidase inhibitors and, less commonly, colesevelam and bromocriptine.

DPP-4 Inhibitors

When food enters the stomach, it triggers the release of GLP-1 by cells in the small intestine. As we said above, this hormone stimulates the secretion of insulin. A class of drugs known as DPP-4 inhibitors delay the inactivation of GLP-1, thereby allowing it to have a more sustained effect. They work in a similar way to GLP-1 receptor agonists but are not quite as good at lowering glucose and have no benefit in reducing body weight or cardiovascular risk.

Sulfonylureas

Sulfonylureas are another class of medications that lower glucose by stimulating insulin secretion from the pancreas. They were discovered in 1942 by a French chemist Marcel Janbon and colleagues, who noticed that patients with typhoid fever treated with a sulfa drug developed hypoglycemia. About ten years later, the first generation of these sulfonamide derivatives were approved for clinical use.

Newer forms of these are still used today. However, unlike GLP-1 receptor agonists and DPP-4 inhibitors, sulfonylureas stimulate insulin secretion by the pancreas no matter how much glucose is present, i.e., their action is not glucose-dependent. This means, unfortunately, that they can cause hypoglycemia.

For many years, these drugs have been used in combination with metformin to lower glucose, and because there are generic forms of sulfonylureas and metformin, they are the cheapest drugs available for the treatment of type 2 diabetes throughout the world.

> Although sulfonylureas are the cheapest medications available globally for the treatment of type 2 diabetes, as they act in a glucose-independent manner, they are associated with a risk of hypoglycemia.

Thiazolidinediones

Thiazolidinediones are yet another class of medication used to treat diabetes and are available as generics.

These work by helping insulin promote glucose uptake into the cells of the body. Some of their side effects include weight gain and fluid retention. They should be avoided in people who have heart failure. They are, however, effective medications that have a role to play in the treatment of select individuals with type 2 diabetes, and do not cause hypoglycemia when used alone or with metformin.

Alpha-glucosidase inhibitors

Alpha-glucosidase inhibitors are drugs that slow the breakdown of carbohydrates in the intestine.

Carbohydrates need to be broken down to glucose before they can be absorbed into the bloodstream. By delaying this breakdown, these medications lower the rise in glucose after meals and reduce the HbA1c by a modest amount. They are usually taken with each meal. Common side effects include flatulence (gas) and diarrhea.

Colesevelam and Bromocriptine

There are two other medications, originally developed for other conditions, that have mild glucose-lowering effects and have been approved by the US FDA for use in people with type 2 diabetes:

1. **Colesevelam** was originally developed to lower cholesterol and was found to modestly lower glucose by an unknown mechanism. The most common side effect is constipation, which tends to be reduced by easting lots of fiber.
2. **Bromocriptine** was developed initially to treat Parkinson's disease and a type of benign pituitary tumor called a prolactinoma. It works in the brain to help lower insulin resistance and therefore blood glucose levels. Side effects include dizziness, nausea, fatigue, and occasionally nasal congestion.

Current Medication Guidelines

The new guidelines by major diabetes and endocrine organizations around the world were updated in 2021. They now recommend that at least one of the newest classes of medications (GLP-1 receptor agonists or SGLT-2 inhibitors) be used in addition to metformin in people with type 2 diabetes who have established cardiovascular disease or are at high risk for cardiovascular disease, *even if their glucose levels are at goal.* If glucose levels are not at goal, these medications are still preferred today because they confer additional benefits of weight loss and no risk of hypoglycemia.

The guidelines recommending which medications to add to metformin consider efficacy, safety and cardiovascular benefit of the products, but not cost. As stated above, generic versions of some medications are available and are much cheaper than the new medications such as insulin analogs. Prices of medicines vary considerably from country to country but are usually more expensive in the USA. However, there are programs that have been made available by many pharmaceutical companies to assist people who cannot afford their medications, so that they can take them as prescribed and do not have to skip them or take reduced doses. We encourage you to discuss this with your clinician if this may be of support to you.

American Diabetes Association Recommendations (2021)

1. Intensify lifestyle therapy and optimize glycemic control for patients with elevated triglyceride levels (1.7 mmol/L [150.6 mg/dl]) and/or low HDL-c (1.0 mmol/L [88.6 mg/dl] for men; 1.3 mmol/L [115.1 mg/dl] for women).
2. For people of all ages with diabetes and atherosclerotic cardiovascular disease (ASCVD) or 10-year ASCVD risk >20%, high-intensity statin therapy should be added to lifestyle therapy.
3. Use aspirin (75–162 mg/day) as a secondary prevention strategy in those with diabetes and a history of ASCVD.
4. People with blood pressure (BP) >120/80 mmHg should be advised on lifestyle changes to reduce this.
5. People with confirmed office-based BP ≥140/90 mmHg should, in addition to lifestyle therapy, have prompt initiation and timely titration of pharmacological therapy to achieve BP goals.

The American Diabetes Association Guidelines for the Pharmacologic Treatment of Type 2 Diabetes (2021)

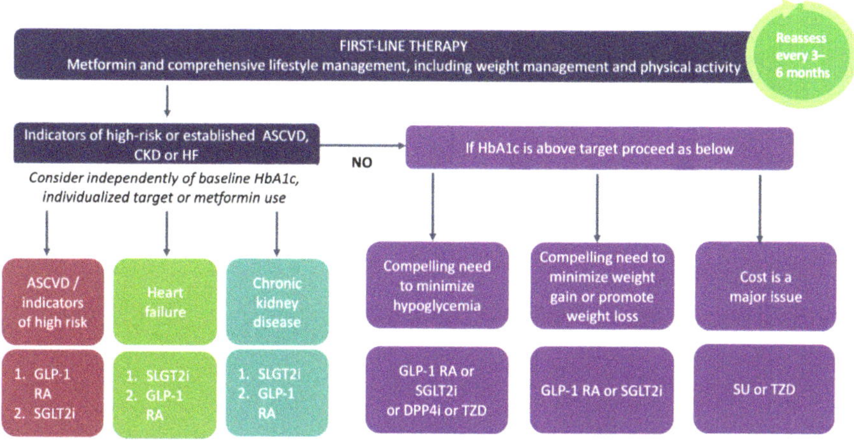

Summary of the American Diabetes Association's guidelines for pharmacologic treatment of type 2 diabetes. *ASCVD, atherosclerotic cardiovascular disease; CKD, chronic kidney disease; HF, heart failure; GLP-1 RA, GLP1 receptor agonists; SGLT2i, SGLT2 inhibitors; DPP4i, Dipeptidyl peptidase-4 inhibitor; TZD, Thiazolidinediones (glitazones); SU, Sulfonylurea.* Adapted from the ASCEND (Academy for Science and Continuing Education in Diabetes and Obesity) Program. http://www.ASCEND-diabetes-obesity.com.

Key Points

- Metformin has some other potential benefits beyond lowering blood sugar levels. It may increase telomere length and favorably affect other cellular markers of ageing.
- Over the past 15 years we have seen new medications come to market that are safer to use, do not cause hypoglycemia, can cause weight loss, and have the added benefit of reducing the risk for cardiovascular disease.
- There are two classes of medications that have been shown to reduce the risk for cardiovascular disease: glucagon-like peptide-1 (GLP-1) receptor agonists and sodium-glucose cotransporter-2 (SGLT-2) inhibitors.

18

BARIATRIC SURGERY

We are in the midst of a burgeoning epidemic of obesity in the United States and in most countries around the world.

Patients with obesity are at a higher risk of developing multiple medical conditions including diabetes, high blood pressure, high cholesterol, many types of cancer, arthritis, sleep apnea and liver disease. Indeed, there's evidence supporting the idea that obesity is the single most important driver of the type 2 diabetes epidemic. Thus, addressing obesity through prevention and treatment holds one of the keys to reducing the personal and population burden of diabetes.

The word bariatric was coined around 1965 from the Greek word *baros*, meaning weight. Bariatric surgery is surgery performed on the stomach and/or intestines to help a person with extreme obesity lose weight. Operations for weight loss work by reducing the capacity of the stomach to accommodate food, altering gut hormone release, and/or producing a form of malabsorption of ingested nutrients.

The three most common types of bariatric surgical procedures are:

1. Gastric bypass.
2. Adjustable gastric band placement.
3. Sleeve gastrectomy.

> At a recent lecture for our Annual Update in Internal Medicine Course, the world-renowned Dr. Daniel Jones, Professor of Surgery at Harvard Medical School, ended his excellent lecture with a little humorous commentary on surgery's (potential) contribution to treating obesity and diabetes. It was a slide with a cartoon depicting two children building sandcastles on the beach. One boy says, "My father is a doctor, and he treats patients with diabetes." The other replies, "My mother is a surgeon, and she cures diabetes"(!)

Most of the time these procedures are performed laparoscopically. The surgical team discuss these options in detail with prospective patients; how they are performed and the pros and cons of each, so that the patient can make an informed decision as to which is most suitable. They also provide multidisciplinary education on nutrition, lifestyle modification, and psychological challenges necessary for a successful outcome. In reality, proper bariatric long-term care means lifelong surveillance.

In the United States, a total of 179,000 surgical procedures were performed in 2013. Five years later, in 2017, 228,000 operations were carried out of which close to 60 % were sleeve gastrectomies.

If you are considering surgery for obesity, an evaluation at the bariatric center will go over the advantages and disadvantages for each of these

Bariatric Surgical Procedures

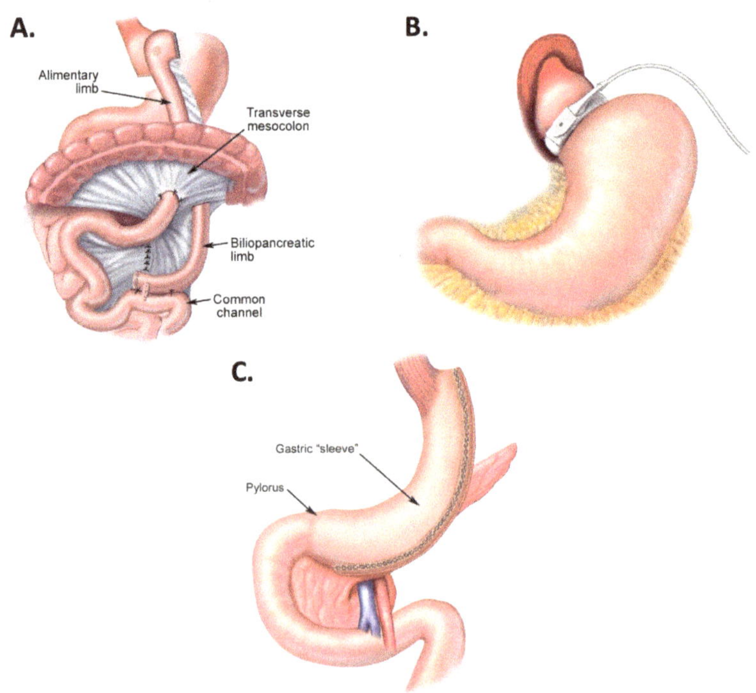

A. Gastric bypass using the 'Roux-en-Y' technique. B. An adjustable gastric band. C. Sleeve gastrectomy. Reproduced with permission from: Jones DB, Torsten A, Schneider B. *Atlas of Metabolic and Weight Loss Surgery*, Cine-Med Publishing, Woodbury, CT, 2010.

operations. In excellent centers, these procedures have a very low mortality ranging from 0.1 to 1 % with the laparoscopic gastric band having the lowest mortality.

Indications for Surgery

> Body Mass Index (BMI) is the standard unit for assessing body weight. It is s a person's weight in kilograms divided by the square of height in meters. There are online calculators you can use, e.g., https://www.cdc.gov/healthyweight/assessing/bmi/adult_bmi/english_bmi_calculator/bmi_calculator.html

Bariatric surgery is typically performed when people with obesity have failed to lose significant weight despite medical measures and have a Body Mass Index (BMI) of either 40 or higher, or a BMI between 35 and 39.9 **and** the person has an associated disease such as type 2 diabetes, high blood pressure or severe sleep apnea or other associated conditions.

Surgery may also be considered even if the BMI in people with type 2 diabetes is between 30 and 34.9 (BMI 27.5 to 32.4 in Asian Americans) if there are multiple comorbid conditions. Bariatric surgery is considered in Asians with a BMI as low as 27.5 with poor control of blood sugar.

Patients considering bariatric surgery are best served by being evaluated at a center that does a high volume of these procedures with a structured and comprehensive evaluation prior to embarking on surgery. Good post-operative care is critically important.

Outcomes

Bariatric surgery can be accompanied by both short-term and delayed complications and is not for everyone. A rigorous screening process is carried out prior to surgery to increase the likelihood of success and well-being in the post-surgical period. The potential complications are discussed with every patient.

Generally, there is a marked improvement in a host of conditions associated with severe obesity following bariatric surgery, including symptoms of gastroesophageal reflux (GERD), arthritis, high blood pressure, heart failure, high cholesterol, diabetes, sleep apnea and liver disease.

Bariatric surgery can also result in significant cost savings. Indeed, the reduction or discontinuation of many prescription drugs following bariatric surgery is remarkable and it has been calculated that as a result the procedure pays for itself within two years of surgery. However, one also needs to consider the potential complications from the surgery.

In the long term, bariatric surgery can produce significant cost savings. Indeed, the reduction or discontinuation of many prescription drugs following bariatric surgery in many people is remarkable and it has been calculated that as a result the procedure pays for itself within two years of surgery.

Bariatric Surgery and Diabetes – the Evidence

Let us now look at the benefits of bariatric surgery for type 2 diabetes. The first report of the effect of bariatric surgery was published in the *Annals of Surgery* in 1987 by Walter Pories and colleagues. They analyzed the results of "identical standardized Greenville Gastric Bypass" surgery in 397 morbidly obese patients, 36% of whom had diabetes or prediabetes prior to surgery:

- The operative mortality was 0.8%.
- Postoperatively, the patients lost significant weight and the weight loss was maintained six years later.
- There was a marked improvement in blood pressure control, physical and mental well-being and diabetes control.
- One hundred and thirty nine of the 141 patients with abnormal glucose levels achieved normal blood glucose levels within four months of surgery without the need for diabetes medications.

The authors conclude that: "The normalization of glucose metabolism after gastric bypass may not be related solely to weight loss and restriction of caloric intake, but may also be due to the bypass of the antrum and duodenum."

In a systematic review published in the *Journal of the American Medical Association* (JAMA) in 2004, Buchwald and colleagues note that "effective weight loss was achieved by morbidly obese patients after bariatric surgery. A substantial number of patients with diabetes, hypertension, hyperlipidemia and obstructive sleep apnea experienced complete resolution or improvement." Their analysis showed that 76.8 % of 1846 patients experienced complete resolution of their diabetes.

A study published in the *Journal of the American Medical Association*

(JAMA) by Dixon and colleagues in 2008 examined the results of gastric banding in the resolution of type 2 diabetes. Using strict criteria of resolution, they found that 73% had achieved remission two years after surgery. This was accompanied by an intensive lifestyle modification program that the patients had been counselled about. Weight regain after surgery can occur so adherence to the lifestyle modification is very important.

Can Bariatric Surgery Decrease Mortality?

In a *New England Journal of Medicine* article in 2007, investigators reported that bariatric surgery was associated with a 40% decrease in mortality in people with severe obesity at the end of 7 seven years! Furthermore, there was a significant decrease in risk for the development of type 2 diabetes in individuals who did not have diabetes at the time of their bariatric surgery.

Endoscopic Surgery

In addition to surgical procedures there are novel endoscopic techniques that have been explored as an alternative to surgery to promote weight loss. One approach is the deployment of a saline filled silicone balloon in the stomach. This induces weight loss by making the person feel fuller faster, hence limiting the amount of food eaten.

Another approach is using heat to resurface the lining of the first part of the small intestine, called the duodenum. This is also done endoscopically as an outpatient procedure. It is referred to as duodenal mucosal resurfacing (DMR) treatment. Preliminary studies have shown that this procedure lowers blood glucose levels and the amount of fat in the liver in people with type 2 diabetes and fatty liver disease. The treatment is commercially available in the United Kingdom.

Patient Stories: Why Didn't I Do This Sooner?

One of us first saw CJ, a Caucasian man who worked in real estate, in consultation in 1999 for management of newly diagnosed type 2 diabetes. At that time, he was 45 years old and commented that he had slowly gained weight since the age of 21, despite regular exercise and trying many different diets which had a yo-yo effect on his weight. He would lose weight but then gain it all back, and some more, and was most frustrated. His wife complained of his snoring and a sleep study confirmed that he had moderate sleep apnea.

At the initial visit he was found to be 70.5 inches [1.79 m] tall and weighed 240 pounds [109 kg]. His calculated BMI was therefore 34 kg/m^2. His blood pressure was normal and clinical examination showed no evidence of any complications of diabetes. His fasting glucose was 170 mg/dL [9.4 mmol/L] and his HbA1c was 9.5%. He was not taking any medications. He was started on metformin, referred to a nutritionist and also recruited a personal trainer.

Despite these efforts, his glucose control remained suboptimal and over the next four years he required more medications, including insulin. I recommended bariatric surgery as an effective treatment option, and we discussed the pros and cons in detail at many visits. I felt strongly that he needed to feel empowered and make the final decision himself. He received material written for patients about surgery for obesity and type 2 diabetes.

Eventually, eight years after being seen initially, he opted to undergo bariatric surgery. He was now 53 years of age, still had no complications of diabetes, but had developed hypertension. His weight was now 280 pounds [127 kg] and he was taking insulin, metformin, a sulfonylurea and a GLP-1 receptor agonist to treat his diabetes. His HbA1c had gradually come down from 9.5% to 7.6%, significantly over the aim of less than 7%. And he was taking all of these diabetes medications, plus a medication for hypertension and a cholesterol lowering drug too....

In 2008, he underwent a Roux-en-Y gastric bypass procedure. There were no complications, and he was discharged from hospital 48 hour after surgery. Within 1 month, he had lost 35 pounds [15.9 kg] and had stopped all of his diabetes medications except for metformin. Six months later, he had lost an additional 15 pounds [6.8 kg] and his HbA1c was now 5.9%!

Over the years he has done well – his weight has now stabilized at 202 pounds [91.6 kg] (almost 80 pounds weight loss!) and his HbA1c has remained stable at 6%. He continues to take only metformin for his diabetes. And – to his wife's relief – his sleep apnea has resolved!

When I saw him one month after surgery, he commented "Why did I wait so long to have this done?! My life is so much better now." And every time I see him, he repeats this lament and expresses his gratitude to me and the team involved with his bariatric surgery.

Take-Home Messages

- Bariatric surgery is a very commonly performed operation and, in good hands, has an inordinately low mortality.
- It is now recommended as part of the treatment of type 2 diabetes and obesity when non-surgical strategies to incur weight loss fail to achieve appropriate goals.
- There are additional benefits in that bariatric surgery can lead to improvement of other associated medical disorders, such as high blood pressure, gastroesophageal reflux disease, hyperlipidemia, osteoarthritis and sleep apnea.

Key Points

- Patients considering bariatric surgery are best served by being evaluated at a center that does a high volume of these procedures with a structured and comprehensive evaluation prior to embarking on surgery. Good post-operative care is critically important.
- A study published in the *Journal of the American Medical Association* (JAMA) by Dixon and colleagues in 2008 examined the results of gastric banding in the resolution of Type 2 diabetes. They noted (using strict criteria to define resolution) that two years after surgery 73% had achieved remission.
- In a *New England Journal of Medicine* article in 2007, the authors reported that bariatric surgery was associated with a 40% decrease in mortality in people with severe obesity at the end of seven years!

19

DIABETES TECHNOLOGY

...I hope advances in machine learning and smart insulins can provide better treatment until a biological cure comes to light...

—S.W., diagnosed T1DM in 2006, *Nature Medicine*, Vol 27, 2021

The common theme is that diabetes technologies such as blood glucose meters, CGM systems, numerous smartphone applications (apps), and insulin delivery systems have tremendous upsides, but also have implementation challenges.

—Mansur Shomali, MD, in *Diabetes Care* special issue on diabetes technology, 2020

Major advances over the last 40 years in both home glucose monitoring and insulin delivery systems have transformed diabetes care. Undoubtedly, further advances in technology, perhaps even incorporating artificial intelligence, will see the light of day in the coming years. This chapter will deal with both topics which we call "diabetes technology."

Self-Monitoring of Blood Glucose (SMBG)

Many people ask about the need for or value of self-monitoring of blood glucose. Measuring your blood glucose at different times of the day provides valuable information regarding the effect of different foods, impact of exercise, and of course, the glucose-lowering efficacy of medications. Many people feel empowered that they can make decisions to optimize blood glucose control based on this information.

Let's now discuss home glucose monitoring systems. There are two major ways for a person with diabetes to measure their own blood glucose: fingerstick glucose testing and continuous glucose monitoring (CGM).

Fingerstick glucose testing

Fingerstick glucoses are obtained by pricking the finger with a small needle, drawing a tiny drop of blood onto a strip which is coated with a special enzyme to measure the glucose. The strip is then attached to a meter which measures the blood glucose concentration using a chemical reaction.

Continuous glucose monitoring

Continuous glucose monitoring systems measure glucose levels continuously by sensors applied to the skin that measure the glucose concentration in interstitial fluid (the fluid between cells) just beneath the skin. These sensors are worn for 10 to 14 days at a time and then replaced. There is another type of sensor that is implanted underneath the skin by a small incision, and which lasts for three months. CGM systems can scan in real-time or intermittently.

> Modern CGM devices communicate with pumps using Bluetooth technology. Some pumps are embedded with software that mean it can automatically respond to the transmitted CGM data with the appropriate rate of insulin infusion.

Real-time CGM systems measure glucose levels continuously, and display the glucose levels on a receiver, smart phone or smart watch in real time. These systems provide alarms and alerts when glucose levels reach certain mutually agreed levels that are considered too high or low for that individual, or when glucose levels rise or fall too fast.

Intermittently scanning CGM systems measure glucose levels continuously, but the levels are only viewed when the user "swipes" the sensor with a reader device or app on a smart phone. Cloud-based technology now also enables the user to share his or her glucose data with others, including healthcare professionals. This is particularly valuable for parents of children who have type 1 diabetes.

Who Should Monitor Glucose Levels and How Often Should They Be Tested?

The frequency with which we recommend blood glucose monitoring depends on the type of diabetes you have, and the types of medications you are taking.

Glucose Monitoring in Type 1 Diabetes

In general, every person with type 1 diabetes should measure glucose levels frequently. We usually recommend that people with type 1 diabetes who use the multiple daily injection regimen and take both long-acting (basal) insulin and rapid-acting (prandial) insulin with meals, should check levels before each meal, before bed, and before certain activities such as exercise or driving, and sometimes two hours after a meal. This means testing six to ten times a day. Since the advent of CGM devices, we believe that they are preferable to fingerstick glucose monitoring, as they provide much more information without the need to frequently prick the finger.

Many newer CGM systems do even not require fingerstick testing to calibrate or standardize the CGM. The only time you would have to prick your finger would be on the rare occasions where you suspect an inaccurate reading that needs double-checking.

Continuous glucose monitoring results in improved HbA1c and reduced rates of low blood glucose (hypoglycemia) in adults with type 1 diabetes. This information was first published in the *New England Journal of Medicine* in a study funded by the Juvenile Diabetes Research Foundation in 2008. In another study published in the *Annals of Internal Medicine*, CGM was shown to improve HbA1c in people with type 2 diabetes who take multiple shots of insulin.

Glucose Monitoring in Type 2 Diabetes

For people who have type 2 diabetes, recommendations regarding blood glucose monitoring vary, depending upon the complexity of the treatment regimen. For example, for people who manage the diabetes with just diet and exercise or perhaps with a medication like metformin, the need to monitor glucose is less essential. Glucose monitoring can, however, provide feedback regarding behaviors, e.g., the impact of certain foods on blood glucose levels, or the

> Glucose monitoring is certainly recommended for people who take medications, such as insulin or sulfonylureas, that may cause hypoglycemia.

effect of exercise on glucose. This can help the individual figure out which diet and exercise options are most effective for their glucose control, and it encourages long-term commitment to recommended lifestyle changes.

Glucose monitoring is certainly recommended for people who take medications, such as insulin or sulfonylureas, that may cause hypoglycemia. We usually recommend measuring glucose at least once a day, usually in the morning before breakfast, particularly for people taking a once-daily injection of basal insulin. In this situation, the dose of the basal insulin is determined by the fasting glucose level.

For people not using insulin but who are taking two or more other medications, we also recommend glucose monitoring once a day or three times per week. Glucose monitoring in these situations does not necessarily improve HbA1c but does provide valuable information about the effects of diet and exercise on glucose levels and makes it easier to adjust doses of medications more appropriately. Once again, this is particularly important if you are taking a medication that may cause hypoglycemia.

In addition to testing glucose in the morning we recommend occasionally testing two hours after meals to determine the impact of the food eaten on glucose levels. We also recommend testing if at any time symptoms of hypoglycemia are experienced.

For people who take medications that do not cause hypoglycemia when used alone or in conjunction with each other – i.e., metformin, DPP-4 inhibitors, GLP-1 receptor agonists, SGLT-2 inhibitors and thiazolidinediones – blood glucose monitoring is not essential but is still recommended. The frequency of blood glucose monitoring is a topic that needs to be discussed between the patient and the health care provider.

For people with type 2 diabetes who take multiple shots of insulin, measuring glucose frequently with either fingerstick glucose devices or CGM is recommended just as we recommend for people with type 1 diabetes who are taking multiple shots of insulin.

Glucose Meters

In the United States, it is important to use glucose meters that have been approved by the Food and Drug Administration (FDA), since the FDA has validated that the meters maintain a high standard of accuracy. It is also important to remember that glucose testing strips have an expiry date, and out-of-date strips should not be used as the readings will be unreliable.

The cost of glucose monitoring meters and strips are covered by all insurance carriers for people with type 1 and type 2 diabetes. CGM devices are covered by commercial insurance for all people with type 1 diabetes who are taking multiple shots of insulin. Medicare (Federal health insurance for people 65 years or older in the USA) covers people with type 1 and type 2 diabetes who fulfill these criteria but not all commercial insurers cover the cost of CGM for people with type 2 diabetes on multiple shots of insulin.

Finally, some substances may interfere with some glucose reading strips. These include acetaminophen and ascorbic acid (vitamin C). If you take either of these medications, you should ensure you choose both a device and strips that are not affected by them.

Insulin Delivery Devices

There have been major advances in the ways insulin can be delivered.

Insulin Pens

Insulin pens have been around for just over 30 years. They are disposable and non-disposable pen-shaped devices containing insulin that is administered by first "dialing" the number of units required, then injecting into the subcutaneous tissue using a very small needle at the end of the pen. These needles are replaced after each use and the pen reused until the insulin is used up. They are certainly more convenient than a vial and syringe and are also more accurate.

Insulin Pumps

Insulin pumps are devices that continuously deliver insulin and enable the user to give doses (referred to as a "bolus dose") to cover meals. Only rapid-acting insulin is used in the pumps. There is no need for long-acting insulin, since the rapid-acting insulin is being delivered continuously throughout the day and night via a small needle that is inserted under the skin and held in place by an adhesive.

There are two main types of pumps. One type uses tubing to deliver the insulin subcutaneously through a small tubing or needle (cannula), the other type of pump attaches directly to the skin without any tubing.

Automated Monitoring-Delivery Systems

Modern CGM devices communicate with pumps using Bluetooth technology. Some pumps are embedded with software that uses this data (including the rate of glucose's rise and fall) to enable the pumps to automatically change the rate of administration of the basal insulin. These are called **sensor-augmented pumps** or **hybrid closed-loop insulin delivery systems**.

When glucose levels drop rapidly or below a certain value, the pump stops delivering insulin until glucose levels rise again, preventing serious hypoglycemia. Similarly, when glucose levels rise too rapidly or reach a certain height, the pump automatically increases the basal insulin infusion rate.

Someone using this type of pump must still administer bolus doses of insulin at meals proportional to the amount of carbohydrate being eaten. A successful "artificial pancreas" would be a completely closed-

An Insulin Infusion Pump With Continuous Glucose Monitoring (CGM)

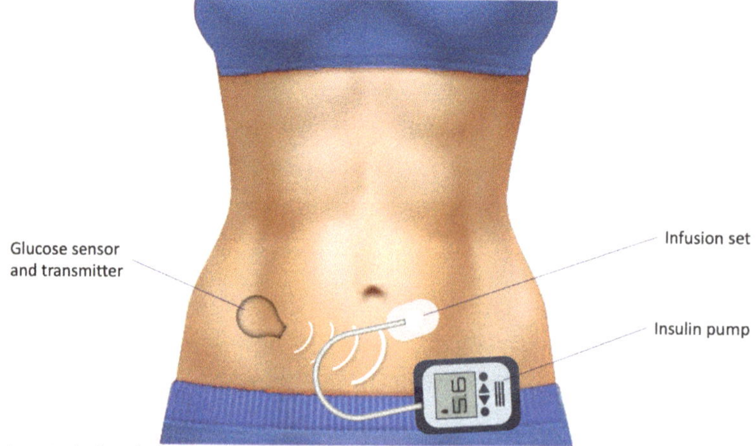

In a 'a hybrid closed-loop system,' the glucose data is transmitted to the pump, which uses software to adjust the basal insulin infusion to increase or decrease as needed.

loop system in which insulin administration is entirely automated, based on glucose readings throughout the day, before and after meals, etc. These are not yet clinically available. However, clinical trials of completely automated devices are underway and preliminary results are promising. It is likely such devices will be available within the next five years.

Patient Stories: Glucose Monitoring and Record Keeping

JG is a 55-year-old woman who had had type 2 diabetes for six years when one of us first saw her. She also has hypertension and an elevated cholesterol (hyperlipidemia) but has no known cardiovascular disease. She has no visual symptoms, but at a recent dilated eye exam she was found to have mild non-proliferative diabetic retinopathy. She has no other complications of diabetes.

She was referred by her primary care physician because her morning glucose readings were around 150 mg/dL [8.3 mmol/L] and her HbA1c was 8.2%. Her physician felt that she might need insulin as the next step in her management. She was already taking two medications for her diabetes - metformin and a sulfonylurea - as well as treatment for her hypertension and elevated cholesterol.

After the initial diagnosis of type 2 diabetes, she started a regular exercise program and lost 10 pounds [4.5 kg], began taking metformin and her HbA1c dropped from 8.5% to 6.5% within six months. A year later, her HbA1c rose again despite her continuing to carefully watch her carbohydrate intake and her regular exercise. A second diabetes medication - a sulfonylurea - was added when her HbA1c rose to 7.5%. Thereafter, the HbA1c came down and remained below 7% for another few years, but six months ago, it rose again. Her weight had not changed - she weighed 165 pounds [74.8 kg] and was 5'4" [1.65 m] giving her a BMI of 28 kg/m^2 (classified as "overweight"). Her blood pressure was well controlled (125/80 mm Hg).

When JG was seen she expressed frustration that her glucose control was worse than she would have liked even though she had continued to walk for 30–40 minutes at least four days a week and also used resistance bands for strength training at least twice a week. She had not altered her diet in any way and took all of her medications every day as prescribed. "Why are my sugars going up now?" she asked, "I do the right things and my HbA1c just goes up!", she said expressing frustration. "I am not really keen to take insulin just yet..." she added.

Indeed, a repeat HbA1c that day was 8.5% and her fasting glucose in the office was 155 mg/dL [8.6 mmol/L]. We explained to her that her situation is common in people with type 2 diabetes and that this had nothing to do with her behavior or adherence to diet, exercise or taking medications. Type 2 diabetes is a "progressive disease." What does this mean? This means that over time the amount of insulin produced by the pancreas decreases, and people need more medications to achieve good control their blood glucose.

"So, what should I do now?", she asked. After some discussion it was suggested that she collect more data for us so we could make some rational suggestions regarding what additional medication might be most appropriate for her. We asked her to test her glucose at home twice a day for one week, testing at different times of the day each day, both before and two hours after meals. For example, test glucose before and two hours after breakfast on Monday, before breakfast and after two hours after lunch on Tuesday, and before breakfast and two hours after dinner on Wednesday. We also asked her to note what she had eaten or what activity she had done on in the two days prior to her next visit, which was scheduled for the following week.

The following week she returned with this information (glucose readings are in mg/dL – divide by 18 to convert to mmol/L):

	Before breakfast	Before lunch	Before dinner	Before bed
Monday	145	186		
Tuesday	155		178	
Wednesday	149			216*
Thursday	164	195		
Friday	149		178	
Saturday	152			238**
Sunday	158		156***	

* Ate out – had fish with a cup of rice and small ice cream.
**Ate out again – had pasta for dinner.
*** Went for an hour's walk after lunch.

This information enabled us to interpret the glucose readings that were obtained with JG. She saw the connection between the amount of carbohydrate she had eaten at dinner on Wednesday and Saturday, and the impact of exercise on her glucose reading after lunch on Sunday. Her morning glucose levels, taken before eating breakfast on waking, were all above goal (usually 80 to 130 mg/dL [4.4–7.2 mmol/L]), and most of her glucose levels after meals were above 180 mg/dL [10 mmol/L].

Based on this information we decided together that the most appropriate medication to add to her treatment would be an injection of a GLP-1 receptor agonist once a week, which would help lower both her morning glucose levels AND glucose levels after meals.

JG started this treatment, and fortunately had no side effects of therapy. Three months later she returned for a follow-up visit much happier and announced, "Not only are my glucose readings better, but I've also lost 5 pounds!" Indeed, her morning glucose readings were now all below 130 mg/dL [7.2 mmol/L] and ranged from 85 to 125 mg/dL [4.7–6.9 mmol/L]; and a few tests that she did two hours after meals were in the 160 to 180 mg/dL [8.9–10 mmol/L] range. Her repeat HbA1c was now 7.1%.

Take-Home Messages

- People with type 2 diabetes have a progressive disease that often requires additional therapy over time. This is because the pancreas gradually produces less and less insulin. And so, when our patients ask, "Will I ever need insulin?", the answer is, "yes, likely." This is not because of a lack of adherence to treatment, but because of the natural history of the disease. In fact, for many people, insulin will be required to maintain good glucose control. So, If you need to start insulin to maintain good glucose control, don't delay!
- Keeping a log of glucose readings and annotating food and exercise is very helpful. It can help people understand the impact of diet and exercise on glucose levels and allow clinicians to make rational choices of medications to help improve glucose control.

Patient Stories: Type 2 or Type 1?

BE was 47 years old when we first met some years ago in 2011. He had been diagnosed with diabetes about 1 week before seeing one of us. One Friday afternoon, he went to see his primary care physician for a routine checkup and was feeling well but commented that he had been getting up to go the bathroom at night for the past few months. His primary care physician did some routine blood tests and called him later that same day, saying, " I don't really know what's going on, but your blood sugar is 846 mg/dL [47 mmol/L]! You better go to the Emergency Room (ER) where they can check on this and treat you!"

As it happens, BE is a nurse who works in the ER, so he drove himself to the ER, where his glucose was found to be 750 mg/dL [41.7 mmol/L].

He was given some intravenous fluids and some insulin to bring the glucose down. He called his doctor who told him he thought he had type 2 diabetes, suggested he start metformin and arranged a follow-up appointment the following week. The ER physician wanted him to go to the hospital's intensive care unit (ICU), but our patient refused, saying "I am a nurse. I will check my glucose at home and report back if there are any problems." So, he went home!

He spent the weekend thinking about his diagnosis and felt that the diagnosis was not correct. He was a very active person, worked three jobs (policeman, ER nurse and school bus driver), exercised most days of the week and was not obese. Plus, there was no family history of diabetes. How could he have type 2 diabetes?! Surely this was type 1! He started his metformin as prescribed but sought specialist opinion and that led to one of us seeing him six days after his initial diagnosis.

When BE came into the exam room, he was really anxious and very stressed. He relayed all his concerns about having diabetes and getting all the complications of the disease.

As stated, he had been in good health, other than being diagnosed with an underactive thyroid (hypothyroidism) as a teenager. He had been maintained on thyroid hormone replacement therapy and his thyroid tests were normal.

His examination was entirely normal. His weight was 172 pounds [78 kg] and height 5'7" [1.7 m] giving him a BMI of 27 kg/m^2. His HbA1c at that time was 12.1%. All his other routine tests, including thyroid function tests, were normal. We took a blood sample to send away for a type 1 diabetes test, which looks for the presence of the antibodies that destroy the insulin-producing pancreatic beta cells

We spent a lot of time talking about the diagnosis and agreed with him that this was almost certainly type 1 diabetes. We also reassured him that if he maintained good glucose control the risks for developing complications were minimal, and that he would be able to lead a totally normal life, continuing to do all that he was currently doing. A reassured patient went home that day feeling a lot more relieved.

His test for type 1 came back positive, confirming that he had type 1 diabetes. As is the case in many people with newly diagnosed diabetes, he initially only required very small doses of insulin, as there is a "honeymoon phase" when small numbers of beta cells are still producing insulin. But within a month or so, his insulin requirements increased, and he needed to take it with each meal, as well as a daily long-acting insulin, which he accepted readily.

Our patient's story does not end there, however. He decided that he would prefer to use an insulin pump and so, within four months of diagnosis, he was using one, adjusting the dose of insulin at meals based on the amount of carbohydrate he was eating (something which is essential to do if you are using a pump). He was testing his glucose six or more times a day. In addition, he also decided he needed to ramp up his exercise to help maintain good glucose levels. Despite working three jobs, he managed to do this. On some days, he would walk for up to 10 miles and go to the gym to do strength training; on other days he would just do a gym workout and use the treadmill or elliptical machines.

Within three months, his HbA1c was 6.1%, and he has managed to maintain it! Since then, his HbA1c has not gone above 6.8%, and most of the time it is less than 6.5%. When CGM became available he started using it, and now he is using a CGM that communicates with his pump, enabling the pump to self-adjust insulin infusion rates based on the glucose readings. He still controls the amount of insulin given at meals.

He has no complications of diabetes and ensures that he has all the necessary tests done regularly based on the checklist that we provide at the end of this book (see page 219). He continues to drive the school bus part time, works in the ER on weekends and remains a full-time police officer.

Below is an example of his continuous glucose monitoring data:

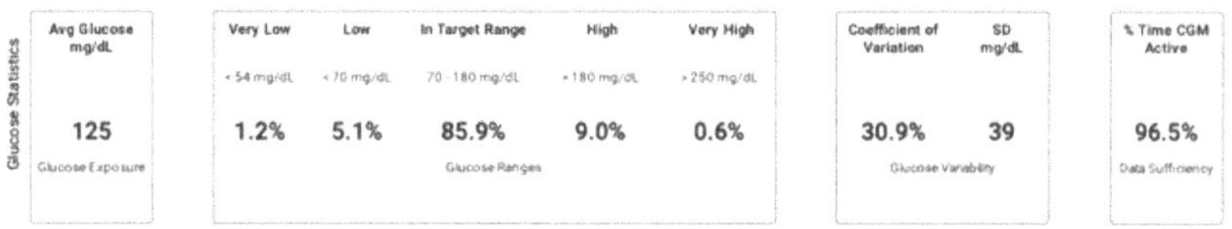

This shows what percent of his glucoses are in range, above 180 mg/dL, or below 70 mg/dL during the past two weeks.

This figure below shows one day of glucose readings – more than 95% of his glucoses are in range between 70 and 180 mg/dL [3.9–10 mmol/L].

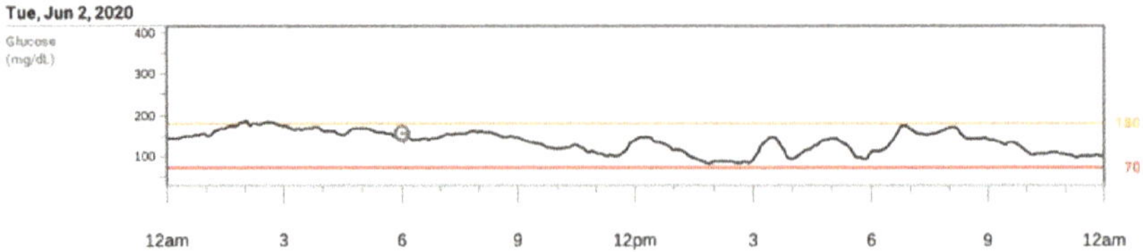

Take-Home Messages

- Some people are misdiagnosed as having type 2 diabetes when they actually have type 1 diabetes.
- People can develop type 1 diabetes at any age. In this case, there were no risk factors for type 2 diabetes other than that he was slightly overweight. He was active, there was no family history of type 2 diabetes and he had had normal lab tests only six months previously (unlike type 1, type 2 less commonly presents acutely).
- If you are diagnosed with type 1 diabetes you can achieve and maintain excellent glucose control and lead a normal life. The advances in technology (newer, more physiological insulins, better insulin delivery systems and continuous glucose monitoring) have made things so much easier for people to maintain good glucose control. But watching what you eat and exercising regularly are equally important.

Patient Stories: Better Living Through CGM

KS is a 56-year-old Caucasian, an entrepreneur, and was initially diagnosed with type 1 diabetes at the age of 41. He has always been very health-conscious and after his diagnosis he made an even more concerted effort to live a healthy lifestyle by exercising daily (both aerobic and strength training) and watching his diet carefully, in particular the amount and type of carbohydrates he ate.

He has been taking four daily injections of insulin daily since diagnosis and testing his glucose six or more times per day. We have had frequent conversations about pumps and more recently continuous glucose monitoring (CGM). His response to using these has been, "I really don't want anything attached to my body. I would rather prick my finger and take multiple injections every day. They don't hurt. I am used to them. And I think I do a pretty good job managing things."

In fact, he has always had good control – his HbA1c levels have never gone above 7.6% and have ranged from 6.8 to 7.6%. He has no complications of diabetes and no other health issues.

Late last year he brought up the subject of CGM spontaneously. "I understand that CGM has really improved recently, that you don't even need to prick your finger to calibrate the device, and that people really love using it. In fact, a good friend of mine, who also has type 1 diabetes and uses CGM, has been bugging me to try it. What have I got to lose? If I don't like it, I will stop using it!"

So, we arranged for KS to obtain a CGM device and he started using it at the beginning of this year. Three months later, he said, "Why did I wait so long to start using this? I guess I am just a slow adopter!" He was delighted with the technology and thought his glucose control was much better now that he could continuously see his glucose levels. Here is an example of his daily glucose profile:

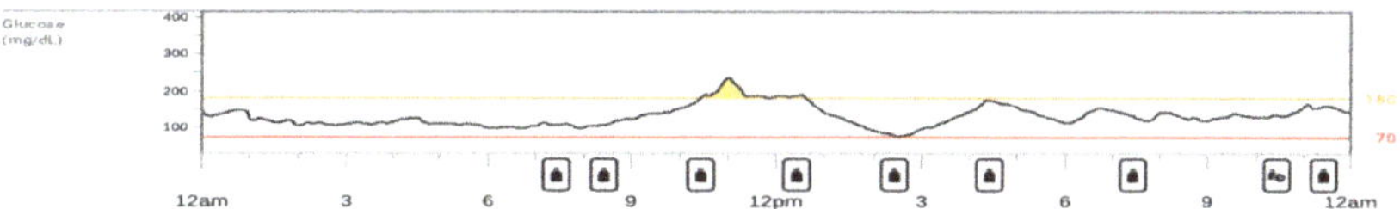

And here are data for his "time in range" – the percentage of time blood glucose levels are in an acceptable range, i.e., between 70–180 mg/dL [3.9–10.0 mmol/L] – during a 3-month period:

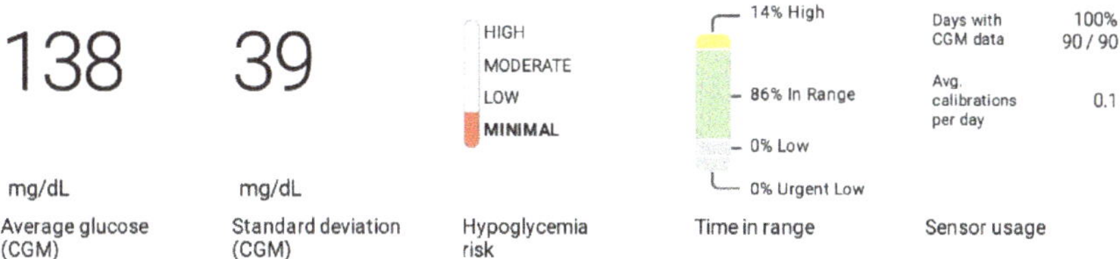

What we see here is that 86% of his glucose readings are in the normal range, only 14% of his glucose levels exceeded this (hyperglycemia), and there were no low glucose readings (no hypoglycemia)!

A repeat HbA1c most recently was a staggering 6.2%! He had achieved this by keeping track of his glucoses, adjusting his carbohydrate intake and insulin dosages in combination with his regular exercise program. And he had not experienced any episodes of hypoglycemia.

Take-Home Messages

- As physicians we can offer people what we consider the best advice, but ultimately the patient makes the decision as whether he or she will adopt these recommendations. We call this "shared decision making."

- Positive feedback is truly the "breakfast of champions." When he saw his HbA1c was 6.2% he was ecstatic and said, "I am totally committed to continuing doing this!"

Patient Stories: Perseverance and Hope!

MJ is a 56-year-old pilot who was diagnosed with type 2 diabetes 14 years ago at the age of 42. He was not overweight, and had no family history of diabetes, so we did tests to determine if he had type 1 diabetes, which were negative.

He was initially treated with oral medications but we both soon realized that despite his relatively low-carbohydrate diet, adhering to a rigorous exercise program, and maintaining a normal weight, he would need insulin to maintain good glucose control. And therein lay the problem, because at the time the Federal Aviation Authority (FAA) would not allow pilots requiring insulin to fly commercial airliners. Since 1996 the FAA has mandated that pilots with insulin-treated diabetes can only be pilot-in-command on private flights, not on commercial flights. The FAA has maintained this regulation whereas some other countries, for example, the United Kingdom and Canada, have begun to allow pilots taking insulin to fly commercial airliners, provided there is a second pilot in the cockpit.

We discussed this problem at length. MJ knew that he needed to start insulin and he also knew that his flying days (at least for a commercial airline) could be over for ever. "I realize this," he said, "but my health is more important, and if I need to be on insulin, I will just have to figure out an alternate plan for my career." So, he started insulin and found a new career path, still in aviation, but behind a desk instead of flight controls, working on behalf of pilots worldwide.

MJ maintained meticulous glucose control. He took long-acting insulin once a day and rapid-acting insulin before meals (four shots per day), adjusted the dose of insulin at meals based on the amount of carbohydrate he was eating and his pre-meal glucose level (we call this **advanced carbohydrate counting**), tested his glucose at least six times a day, and continued to exercise regularly. His HbA1c ranged between 6.3 and 7.2%, and he had no episodes of hypoglycemia. Every year, we would write the appropriate letters to the FAA stating how well-controlled he was, filled out the appropriate forms applying for reinstatement of his commercial pilot's medical certificate, and hoped that he would receive positive news from the FAA. And every year the application was resubmitted, and the response remained unfavorable.

The concern that the FAA outlined was that a pilot with diabetes may experience episodes of high or low blood sugar during a flight, and this could potentially result in an emergency if the pilot lost control of the aircraft. The FAA thus deemed it too risky to allow pilots with insulin-treated diabetes to control a commercial aircraft.

But slowly thing started to change. More pilots lobbied to get their licenses reinstated. Organizations like the American Diabetes Association proposed a set of rigorous guidelines that pilots needed to meet in order to apply to fly commercially again. Slowly but surely the FAA came around to agreeing to review each case individually.

Pilots brought lawsuits against the FAA in the hope that the organization would publish a set of achievable standards on which to base their decision. In a court filing the FAA stated, "A hypoglycemic event, which can result in impaired cognitive function, seizures, unconsciousness, and even death, that occurs in the cockpit of a commercial flight has the potential to place the safety of hundreds of individuals in jeopardy."

But ultimately, the FAA changed its mind. In a court filing in October 2019, the FAA now stated, "Recent advances in technology and diabetes medical science have allowed the FAA to develop an evidence-based protocol that can both identify a subset of low-risk applicants whose glycemic stability is sufficiently controlled and also ensure these pilots can safely maintain diabetic control for the duration of a commercial flight," wrote the Federal Air Surgeon, Michael Berry.

We resubmitted the application for MJ to fly commercially. We once again confirmed that his glucose control was meticulous (by this stage he was using CGM), that almost 90% of his glucose readings were in the normal range, that the remainder were all less than 250 mg/dL [13.9 mmol/L] and that he had not experienced any episodes of hypoglycemia, easily surpassing the FAA criteria for reinstatement of his commercial airline license. Three months later, a day before his birthday, and a day before his general pilot's license was due to expire, MJ reached out to me. "We won!", he said. He had received approval from the FAA to fly commercially again!

Ever since he was a boy, he said, his "only dream was to fly planes." He had been living his dream and then it was dashed by diabetes, but now, thanks to scientific and technological advances, he was once again soaring in the sky and living his dream.

Take-Home Message

Individuals taking insulin and utilizing technological advances can conquer many challenges – both personal and those imposed by regulatory agencies and live a full and fulfilling life.

Key Points

- Continuous glucose monitoring has been shown to improve HbA1c and reduce rates of hypoglycemia in adults with type 1 diabetes.
- Current CGM devices communicate with pumps using Bluetooth technology. Some pumps are embedded with software that can use these data (as well as the rate of rise and fall of glucose) which then enables the pumps to automatically change the rate of infusion of the basal insulin.
- For some individuals the quick and easy feedback from a CGM device empowers them to make wise and rational choices about adjusting their diet, exercise and medication regimen.

20

DIABETES IN PREGNANCY

A mother is always the beginning. She is how things begin.

—Amy Tan

This chapter will discuss the important topic of managing diabetes in pregnancy. There are two clinical situations in which this is relevant:

1. Women who are known to have diabetes prior to becoming pregnant (pre-gestational or **pre-existing diabetes**), and
2. Women who develop diabetes during pregnancy (**gestational diabetes**).

Managing diabetes during pregnancy should be undertaken by clinicians who are experienced in this field and who conduct close and frequent follow-ups.

Pre-existing Diabetes

A successful pregnancy is possible for most women with pre-existing diabetes. Excellent glucose control is vitally important, with normal or close to normal blood glucose levels, before, during and after the pregnancy. This is necessary for the health of the mother, the fetus, and the newborn baby.

> Women with diabetes who maintain excellent glucose control during the first trimester do not have any increased risk of any fetal congenital abnormalities.

Glucose Control

We have known for many years that poor glucose control prior to a pregnancy means that glucose control is also likely to be poor for most of the first trimester. This is an important time for fetal formation and development, since high glucose levels in the mother cross the placenta and increase the risk for major congenital malformations. The reason for this is unknown.

On the other hand, we know that good glucose control prior to and during this important time of fetal development reduces the risk for these congenital anomalies significantly. In fact, women with diabetes who maintain excellent glucose control during the first trimester do not have any increased risk of any fetal congenital abnormalities compared to women without diabetes.

High glucose levels in the second and third trimesters of pregnancy are also associated with developmental problems:

- The high maternal glucose levels cross the placenta and stimulate the fetus' pancreas to produce too much insulin.
- Insulin acts like a growth factor and thus this excessive insulin results in excessive growth of the fetus, a condition we call **macrosomia**.
- This in turn may lead to premature delivery of a larger than normal baby.
- Large newborns may have difficulty breathing due to their immature lungs. It may also suffer from low glucose levels (hypoglycemia) as, after delivery, its immature pancreas continues to produce increased levels of insulin.
- Large babies can have mechanical difficulties at delivery and often require a cesarean section.

Once again, keeping glucose levels close to or normal during this part of the pregnancy significantly lowers these risks, the result being the delivery of a neonate with none of these complications.

Insulin

Insulin treatment is safe during pregnancy and is the treatment of choice before and during pregnancy. Women who become pregnant should expect their insulin requirements to change during the pregnancy. Initially, insulin requirements may decrease in the first trimester, but during the second and third trimesters there is a need to take more insulin to maintain good glucose control. Following delivery, however, there is a sudden predictable decrease in insulin requirements.

Ideal Glucose Levels

The goals for glucose levels in pregnancy differ from those in non-pregnant adults. This is because even in normal pregnancies glucose levels tend to be lower than they are in the non-pregnant state.

We recommend that women who are pregnant achieve an HbA1c of less than 6%, if this can be done without increasing the risk of hypoglycemia, or as close as possible to 6%. In addition, we recommend that fasting glucose levels be less than 95 mg/dL [5.3 mmol/L]. Glucose levels one and two hours after meals should be less than 140 [7.8] and less than 120 mg/dL [6.7 mmol/L], respectively. Women with pregestational diabetes should monitor their glucose levels before and one or two hours after each meal, and before bed. Alternatively, use of continuous glucose monitors is recommended (see page 172).

Any woman with diabetes must plan her pregnancy carefully, be sure that glucose levels are as close to normal as possible prior to conception and be aware of the need to maintain these good glucose levels throughout the pregnancy and following delivery.

Gestational Diabetes

Gestational diabetes is diabetes that first manifests during pregnancy, and usually only occurs after the first trimester, once the fetal organs have been formed. It is common and affects almost 10% of all pregnancies. Because it is common, screening is routine in all pregnancies and is usually undertaken between the 24th and 28th week of pregnancy. If the screening test is abnormal (a glucose of more than 140 mg/dL [7.7 mmol/L]), a more formal glucose tolerance test is undertaken to confirm the diagnosis.

Because gestational diabetes develops after the first trimester, the risk of congenital malformations is not an issue. But, as with pre-gestational diabetes in pregnancy, it can cause:

- Excessive growth of the fetus and premature delivery of a larger than normal baby (macrosomia).
- Associated immaturity of the fetal organs.
- Increased frequency of cesarean section.
- Risk of hypoglycemia after birth.

Women who develop gestational diabetes are initially treated with diet and as much exercise as they can achieve. If this does not result in acceptable glucose levels, insulin therapy is indicated.

Non-insulin Medications

There have been some studies looking at the use of some oral medications for women who develop gestational diabetes. These include metformin and sulfonylureas. While the studies have shown no major safety concerns, it is easier to achieve normal glucose levels with insulin compared to using these medications and thus we prefer to use insulin, which is more widely accepted.

Post-Partum

Women who develop gestational diabetes should have glucose levels checked six weeks after delivery. In most cases, glucose levels have returned to normal by this time. In a small percentage of people, glucose levels remain elevated. However, having gestational diabetes indicates an increased risk for the development of type 2 diabetes in subsequent years.

Up to 50% of women who have gestational diabetes will go on to develop type 2 diabetes in subsequent years. Women who have previously had gestational diabetes and whose glucose levels returned to normal postpartum should be screened earlier in subsequent pregnancies, as the risk for recurrence of gestational diabetes is high.

Prevention

There is evidence that weight loss in women who are overweight or obese prior to any pregnancy reduces the risk for the development of gestational diabetes, and certainly weight loss where appropriate following the pregnancy reduces the risk for the development of type 2 diabetes.

A study published in the *Journal of the American Medical Association* (JAMA) in 2021 showed that in 2529 women who drank up to 2 cups of caffeinated beverages like coffee and tea, there was a 47% reduction in risk for the development of gestational diabetes. Note that this intake did not exceed the recommended intake of caffeine during pregnancy, and it had no other pregnancy-related adverse effects such as preeclampsia.

Patient Stories: A Healthy Baby

RB is a 35-year-old Hispanic woman who was referred for management of diabetes that first manifested in her early third trimester. This was her first pregnancy. Prior to becoming pregnant, she weighed 145 pounds [5.8 kg] and was 5'1" [1.55 m] tall, giving her a BMI of 27 kg/m^2 (overweight). Her ideal body weight is around 125 pounds.

She had been healthy all her life. She exercised regularly and tried to adhere to a healthy diet. She did not smoke or drink any alcohol. She commented that both her parents and maternal grandmother had diabetes and were taking medications for this but did not require insulin. She had an older sister who also had gestational diabetes diagnosed during her second pregnancy.

As part of routine screening during pregnancy, she had a glucose challenge test at 26 weeks' gestation. The test results showed an abnormally elevated blood glucose level. She subsequently had a formal glucose tolerance test, and this confirmed the diagnosis of gestational diabetes.

When seen by one of us she had a number of concerns: "Will this adversely affect my baby? Will I be able to breast feed? Does this resolve after pregnancy? How should I best manage this now?"

We discussed the need to maintain normal glucose levels for the remainder of her pregnancy to reduce any risks to her baby and reassured her that both she and her baby would be monitored very closely for the remainder of the pregnancy. We also reassured her that there was no contraindication to breast feeding. We advised her that it was highly likely that the diabetes would resolve following the delivery of her baby, but that she was at increased risk for the development of type 2 diabetes over the years. She would need to be tested six weeks after delivery to confirm that the diabetes had gone away. Following that, she would need an annual screening test for diabetes.

She was referred to a nutritionist and diabetes nurse educator and started testing her glucose multiple times a day, including before and 1 hour after eating. Glucose goals were discussed with her. She was advised that if she could not achieve these goals with diet and exercise, she would require insulin.

She did extremely well and did not require insulin. She delivered a healthy 7-pound baby boy at 38 weeks' gestation. Six weeks after delivery, her glucose test was normal. She subsequently worked on a weight loss program. Her baby boy is now three years old, and her glucose levels remain normal. She is keen to have another child and both the obstetrician and endocrinologist have told her to proceed. We advised her that there is a high probability (30 to 70% chance) that she will once again develop gestational diabetes and that she should be screened earlier than 24 weeks in her next pregnancy.

Take-Home Messages

- A strong family history of type 2 diabetes and being overweight puts one at a higher risk for the development of gestational diabetes.
- Managed appropriately, gestational diabetes is associated with excellent outcomes for both mother and baby.
- If a woman has gestational diabetes during one pregnancy, there is a 30 to 70% chance of it recurring in subsequent pregnancies.
- Women with a history of gestational diabetes should be screened annually for the development of type 2 diabetes.

Key Points

- Any woman with diabetes must plan her pregnancy carefully, be sure that glucose levels are as close to normal as possible prior to conception and be aware of the need to maintain these good glucose levels throughout the pregnancy and following delivery.
- Gestational diabetes is common and affects almost 10% of all pregnancies.
- If needed, insulin is the treatment of choice during pregnancy.
- Up to 50% of women who have gestational diabetes will go on to develop type 2 diabetes in subsequent years.

21

COMPLEMENTARY AND ALTERNATIVE MEDICINE

Live in each season as it passes; breathe the air, drink the drink, taste the fruit, and resign yourself to the influence of each.

—Henry David Thoreau

Complementary and alternative medicine (CAM) has been defined as a group of diverse medical and healthcare systems, practices and products that are not normally part of conventional medicine. Another term for this approach is "Integrative Medicine."

Surveys reveal that:

- The use of CAM is widespread amongst patients with diabetes, more so than individuals without diabetes. In one survey more than 85% of people with diabetes had availed of CAM in the past year.
- Its use increases up to 3-fold after diagnosis.
- It is more common in those aged over 65 years, in women and in those with at least a high school education.
- The use of CAM and the type used varies between countries.
- The most common types include dietary supplements, herbal products, cupping and acupuncture.

In this chapter we discuss the major dietary supplements that people with diabetes use and the role of yoga and meditation.

Cinnamon

Cinnamon is a spice obtained from the inner bark of several tree species from the genus *Cinnamomum*. It is commonly used to flavor a wide variety of foods.

Alam Khan and colleagues published a study of cinnamon in the journal *Diabetes Care* in 2003. This was a small study of 60 people, 30 of whom received cinnamon (1, 3 or 6 grams daily) and 30 that received placebo:

- After 40 days, all three of the cinnamon recipients had a significant lowering of fasting blood sugar, LDL cholesterol and triglycerides.
- The more cinnamon consumed, the greater the benefit. Placebo recipients saw no benefit.
- There were no side effects and no problems with compliance were encountered.

However, other studies have **not** shown any significant benefit. The challenges with these studies include the fact that only a small number of patients were studied, different kinds and different doses of cinnamon were used.

It is likely that cinnamon is safe. Caution has been advised in the use of "high doses," namely more than 4 grams a day, as this may cause liver damage or potentially interact unfavorably with certain medications.

Much more rigorous research is needed to answer the question as to whether cinnamon is a good adjunctive supplement for people with diabetes. In the meantime, it is reasonable for a person with diabetes to add cinnamon (1 to 3 grams daily) to their diet for six to eight weeks and see what effect it has on their blood sugar levels. A strategic way to do this would be to add it to the coffee they are drinking; you will also be benefiting from the many health benefits of coffee! (See chapter 5, page 35.)

Can Cinnamon Prevent Diabetes?

A pilot study of 51 people with prediabetes demonstrated that the addition of cinnamon to the diet over a 12-week period led to stabilization of blood glucose levels.

The study was performed by Romeo and colleagues at Joslin Diabetes Center and the Division of Endocrinology at Beth Israel Deaconess Medical Center in Boston and was published in the *Journal of the Endocrine Society* in 2020. The lead author concluded, "These findings provide the rationale for longer and larger studies to address if cinnamon can reduce the risk of developing type 2 diabetes over time."

Bitter Gourd

Bitter gourd (*Momordica charantia*) belongs to the gourd family of plants, along with zucchini, squash, pumpkin, and cucumber. It is an edible vine fruit that grows in the tropics and is a staple in many types of Asian cuisine. It has a long history of use in Asian and African traditional medicines.

Evidence

In a small study published in the *Journal of Ethnopharmacology* in 2018, the authors studied the effect of daily consumption of 2.5 grams of bitter gourd powder over a period of eight weeks. The subjects were 52 individuals from Tanzania with prediabetes. Forty-four participants completed the study and most of their fasting blood sugar levels were found to have fallen modestly. The effect was not seen in all participants but was more pronounced in individuals that had higher baseline blood sugar levels before the treatment.

In another Indian bitter gourd study published in 2017 in the *Journal of Traditional and Complementary Medicine*, the authors studied a total of 30 patients. They noted a significant drop of blood glucose in ten participants receiving bitter gourd. Incidentally, in the same study, a similar effect was seen in another ten people receiving kohlrabi ("knol-khol") juice and no effect was seen in the ten patients receiving ash gourd (winter melon).

This study suffers from having only a few patients enrolled and a limited follow-up. Hence, no generalizations can be made, and no meaningful conclusions can be drawn, and the bitter truth (pun intended) is that we need rigorous, well-designed, statistically powered studies in the future.

Fenugreek

Fenugreek (*Trigonella foenum-graecum*) is an herb like clover native to the Mediterranean region, southern Europe, and western Asia. The seeds are used in cooking, to make medicine, or to hide the taste of other medicine. Fenugreek seeds smell and taste somewhat like maple syrup. Fenugreek leaves are eaten in India as a vegetable.

Evidence

In a study published in the *Journal of Diabetes and Metabolic Disorders* in 2015 the authors addressed whether fenugreek could prevent the development of diabetes in people with pre- diabetes. One hundred and forty people with prediabetes were enrolled in a randomized, 3-

year trial.

Seventy-four participants received 5 grams of a debittered powder of fenugreek twice daily, along with 200 ml of water 30 minutes before meals, and 66 individuals served as controls. Participants were both men and women aged 30 to 70 years.

At baseline and three months follow-up weight, BMI, fasting blood glucose levels, blood glucose levels after eating (postprandial glucose levels), lipid profile and insulin levels were recorded.

The fenugreek participants had lower fasting and postprandial glucose levels, lower LDL cholesterol (bad cholesterol) levels and higher insulin levels. The individuals in the control group were 4.2 times more likely to develop type 2 diabetes compared to those in the fenugreek group.

The fenugreek participants had lower fasting and postprandial glucose levels, lower LDL cholesterol (bad cholesterol) levels and higher insulin levels.

This study is encouraging and needs to be duplicated with a larger number of individuals and a longer follow-up period. Adherence to a supplement that may not be palatable to a significant number of individuals could be a detriment to its widespread use, even if further large-scale scientific studies validate the above results.

A review article in 2017 in the *International Journal of Nutritional, Pharmacological and Neurological Diseases* concluded that fenugreek likely has a stimulating or regenerative effect on beta cells (insulin producing cells) in the pancreas and documented benefits for patients with both type 1 and type 2 diabetes.

An encouraging study into fenugreek's potential to prevent type 2 diabetes found that it resulted in lower fasting and postprandial (after a meal) glucose levels, lower LDL cholesterol (bad cholesterol) levels and higher insulin levels.

Chromium

Chromium is one of the most common elements in the earth's crust and in sea water and exists in several oxidative states.

Interest in chromium and its role in diabetes piqued in the 1970s following an intriguing case report in the *American Journal of Clinical Nutrition* in 1977. A patient on total parenteral nutrition (TPN), where all nutrition is supplied as fluids into the veins, developed severe signs of diabetes with weight loss and high blood sugar levels. Curiously, he did not respond to insulin. Based on some preliminary human studies, he was given supplemental chromium. Over the next two weeks he improved dramatically with lower blood glucose levels and the insulin was discontinued. This observation was subsequently validated in other patients receiving TPN. Now chromium is routinely added to TPN solutions.

These studies inform us that chromium deficiency leads to diabetes but beg the question: Does supplemental chromium benefit glucose control in people with diabetes?

Evidence

In an article published in *Diabetes Care* in 2004, Cefalu and colleagues addressed the role of chromium in health and in diabetes. They concluded that chromium supplementation, especially in the form of chromium picolinate, improves both glucose and insulin metabolism in patients with type 1 and type 2 diabetes and in patients with gestational diabetes.

They further suggest that the previous studies that had shown no benefit had included patients receiving a different form of chromium, sub-optimal dosing of chromium and had included both diabetic and non-diabetic participants.

However, the results of other trials are not so positive, and the scientific community and the lay public await more definitive trials, which would need to include larger numbers of people followed for a reasonably long period of time. But such trials are expensive and need significant funding.

The American Diabetes Association does not currently recommend Chromium supplementation in its nutritional guidelines.

Yoga

Yoga is an ancient practice from India dating back thousands of years that has gained widespread acceptance in the United States and worldwide. Yoga incorporates several elements, notably breathing techniques and physical postures. The latter can be difficult for individuals with severe arthritis, but those with limited flexibility can still do yoga sitting comfortably in a chair (often referred to as "gentle yoga").

Evidence

The published scientific literature on the benefits of yoga is scant.

A study published by Hegde and colleagues in *Diabetes Care* in 2011 looked at 123 patients, divided according to whether or not they had complications, and assigned them to standard care or standard care plus at least 3 yoga sessions per week at a designated yoga center over a 3-month period. Yoga participants had a significant reduction in BMI, blood sugar control and in markers of oxidative stress, which are indicative of damage to cells and tissues.

It is difficult to make a blanket endorsement such as "people with diabetes doing yoga have health benefits," because a small number of patients were included in this study, follow-up was short, and there are many kinds of yoga taught throughout the world.

Of interest is an illuminating article published in *Diabetes Research* in 2016 entitled "Yoga for Adults with Type 2 Diabetes: A Systematic Review of Controlled Trials." The authors examined 25 original studies - 12 randomized control trials and 13 nonrandomized trials - with an aggregate of 2170 participants. The yoga interventions ranged from 15 days to 12 months and varied in practice frequency, content, and intensity.

They concluded that, "Overall the findings suggest that the yoga-based practices may have significant beneficial effects on multiple factors including blood sugar control, lipid levels, body composition and blood pressure." Mood, sleep and quality of life were deemed to have improved in the patients doing yoga. They also concluded that there was a need for additional, rigorous, high quality randomized trials.

Our Approach

We feel that yoga is here to stay. It is generally safe. It is best learned from a trusted instructor. Once learnt, one can do it at home and even when traveling, on the beach or in a hotel room.

> When practicing a "multimodal" approach, including a good diet, exercise regime, weight control and different CAM modalities such as yoga, it can be difficult to pinpoint exactly which aspect is improving a person's glucose control.

We believe it is reasonable for individuals with diabetes to practice yoga, while keeping tabs on their eating habits, weight and blood sugar levels. However, it can be difficult to identify exactly what is improving a person's glucose control when we take this "multimodal" approach, for example, of yoga, drinking coffee, eating mindfully, and exercising more regularly.

Meditation

There are several different kinds of meditation. Transcendental Meditation (TM) is a mantra-based technique practiced by millions of individuals throughout the world.

The authors of a study published in the *Archives of Internal Medicine* in 2006 sought to see the effects of TM on components of metabolic syndrome and coronary heart disease (CHD).

They randomized 103 patients with stable CHD to either 16 weeks of the practice of TM or to standard health education (the control group).

The TM group experienced beneficial changes in blood pressure and insulin resistance when compared to the control group.

The authors concluded that "TM may modulate the physiologic response to stress and improve CHD risk factors."

Other Modalities

Other modalities such as cupping and acupuncture have been used by people with diabetes. Cupping involves the use of heat and glass cup shaped devices to create a suction force on the skin. Of note, it can initially lead to abrasions of the skin and blisters which can then become infected. For these reasons we do not recommend this modality. Acupuncture has been used with some reported efficacy on pain reduction in people with painful peripheral neuropathy.

One of the challenges with these two modalities of treatment is the variability and lack of standardization when they are performed, even within the same jurisdiction. Hence, there is very limited evidence on their effect, for example, on glucose control.

There are now complementary and alternative medical centers in some major academic medical institutions, where funding will allow well-designed, rigorous and scientific studies to be conducted.

Key Points

- Surveys reveal that the use of CAM is widespread amongst patients with diabetes.
- Its use is more prevalent amongst people with diabetes compared to individuals without diabetes. In one survey more than 85% of people with diabetes had availed of CAM in the past year.
- Complementary and alternative medical centers are now established in a limited number of major academic medical institutions, where funding will be available to carry out rigorous and scientifically robust trials.

22

PANCREATIC TRANSPLANTATION

The measure of life is not its duration, but its donation.

—Peter Marshall

The first attempt at pancreatic transplantation was carried out more than half a century ago, in 1966 by Drs. Richard Lillehei and William Kelly. It has now evolved into a procedure where both a pancreas and kidney are transplanted at the same time, known as a Simultaneous Pancreas and Kidney (SPK) transplantation. SPK transplantation is now an established treatment for people with type 1 diabetes who are also suffering from advanced or end-stage renal disease (ESRD).

In the US, there are three types of transplants available for patients with insulin-requiring diabetes:

1. Simultaneous Pancreas Kidney (SPK) transplantation.
2. Pancreas After Kidney (PAK) transplantation.
3. Pancreas Transplantation Alone (PTA).

In the US, more than 75% of transplants are SPK. PTA is primarily done in individuals who have frequent life-threatening episodes of hypoglycemia (low blood glucose).

Simultaneous Pancreas Kidney Transplantation

Indications for SPK transplantation include:

1. Difficult to control blood sugar levels.
2. Frequent insulin reactions with potentially dangerously low blood sugar levels.
3. Concomitant serious kidney disease.

The results of SPK transplantation are most encouraging. In those with type 1 diabetes and kidney failure, transplantation results in a dramatic improvement in their quality of life. Patients no longer need to undergo dialysis and are also freed from having to monitor blood sugar levels, manage blood sugar swings and take insulin. Quite a relief!

Also noteworthy is the survival benefit in these patients when compared with similar patients on chronic dialysis. Studies have shown that survival in SPK transplantation at seven years after surgery is 77%. This is significantly better than the 40% survival in patients who remain on dialysis.

Eighty to 90% of patients have optimal blood sugar levels a year after receiving SPK transplant, and these patients require no insulin.

Other Benefits

There are also other favorable metabolic effects and improvements in health seen with SPK transplantation:

- LDL (bad cholesterol) decreases.
- HDL (good cholesterol) increases.
- Blood triglycerides (a kind of fat in the blood) decrease.
- Diabetic nephropathy (kidney dysfunction) stabilizes.
- Fracture risk in men decreases.
- Reproductive health is restored or maintained (in one report, 47 pregnancies were recorded in 34 SPK transplant recipients and resulted in 38 live and healthy newborns!).

The topic of quality of life after SPK transplantation for the treatment of chronic renal failure in patients with type 1 diabetes has been reviewed by Ziaja and colleagues in the journal *Transplantation Proceedings* in 2009. They found that, compared to kidney transplantation alone (KTA), patients who underwent SPK transplantation had improved well-being, less pain, and both better physical and cognitive function. They concluded that SPK transplantation was associated with a positive overall impact on selected quality of life parameters, compared to KTA, for patients with type 1 diabetes.

Pancreatic Islet Cell Transplantation

Pancreatic islet cell transplantation is a new procedure where a deceased person's pancreas is harvested for islet cells (50-70% of which are the insulin-producing beta cells), which are then injected into the portal vein, a large vein that carries blood into the liver.

It is an exciting new potential therapy for type 1 diabetes but is currently only approved (in the US) for clinical trials. It is usually only performed for people with serious and progressive type 1 diabetes.

In one recent trial, 9 out of 10 recipients had excellent blood sugar control, with no episodes of very low blood sugar, one year after the procedure. Two years after, 4 of the 10 still had similar results and were not needing to take insulin.

Potential Negatives

Potential downsides of islet cell transplantation include:

- Pain, bleeding and blood clots.
- Failure of the procedure.
- Side effects of the medications used to prevent rejection, e.g., increased propensity for infections and increased risk for certain cancers.
- Development of antibodies against the donor cells that might make subsequent organ transplantation challenging.

Key Points

- Eighty to 90% of people have optimal blood sugar levels a year after receiving an SPK transplant and these patients are rendered completely insulin free.
- Survival in SPK transplantation seven years following surgery was 77%. This was significantly better than the 40% survival in the group of patients who remained on dialysis.

23

STEM CELLS AND DIABETES

I think about it (a cure) all the time. I wake up thinking about it. It's a quest that we are not going to give up on.

—Dr. Doug Melton, 2019

The topic of stem cells is of great interest to the medical and scientific community. An excellent review was published by Blau and Daley in the *New England Journal of Medicine* in 2019.

Stem cells are the cells from which other cells with specialized functions arise. Under optimal conditions in the body and in the laboratory, stem cells divide to form more cells, termed daughter cells. These daughter cells either transform into other stem cells (a process called self-renewal) or differentiate into specialized kinds of cells such as brain cells, heart muscle cells, liver cells and so on. Because of this novel attribute, we refer to stem cells as "pluripotent" - they have multiple ("pluri-") potentials in terms of which types of cells they can become.

Stem cells are found in embryos, as the source of all cells, and in adult tissues, where they serve as an "internal repair service." Interestingly, we now know that stem cells can also be derived from "reprogrammed" adult cells. It has been said that life without stem cells would last a mere four weeks.

Promising Research

Stem cell research has four promising ramifications:

1. Understanding the process by which normal specialized cells develop.
2. Understanding the genesis of medical diseases.
3. Use as a tool for the study of the efficacy and safety of new medications.

4. Curing chronic medical disorders. Stem cell therapy is part of what is referred to as "regenerative medicine."

Amongst the major academic stem cell institutes are those at Harvard, Stanford, Yale, and UCLA in the United States and Oxford and Cambridge in the UK. Active stem cell research is also being conducted in Japan, China, and other countries. There are also many companies in the private sector with brilliant scientists working, often collaboratively with academic laboratories, to translate basic science discoveries into practical treatments.

Stem Cells and Diabetes

In type 1 diabetes, the insulin-producing beta cells of the pancreas are destroyed, and patients require insulin injections for the rest of their life.

Stem cells can be coaxed into becoming beta cells. However, one of the challenges with stem cell transplantation in a patient with type 1 diabetes is that the immune system that attacked the beta cells in the first place, will also attack the new beta cells. Researchers are currently working hard to address this problem.

Harvard's Stem Cell Institute

Dr. Doug Melton at Harvard's Stem Cell Institute is on a personal mission. Both his children have type 1 diabetes and he is driven to find a cure. After more than a decade of painstaking research, Melton's laboratory produced beta cells and showed in animal models that they can sense the blood sugar levels and secrete insulin.

The next step will be to develop ingenious ways to protect the transplanted beta cells from being rejected by the transplantee's immune system. Once that is done, rigorous trials in humans will follow to assess the safety and efficacy of stem cell transplantation as a cure for type 1 diabetes. Many experts predicted that this would happen within the next decade. Doug Melton said in 2019, "I think about it [a cure] all the time. I wake up thinking about it. It's a quest that we are not going to give up on."

It is hard to predict when this will come true, but in 2021, Dr. Melton's dedication resulted in a huge leap forward. On June 29th, 2021, Brian

Shelton, a patient with type 1 diabetes who had suffered from life-threatening episodes of severe hypoglycemia, received a stem cell infusion developed by Dr. Melton's team. This resulted in Brian being able to come off insulin, and of course, resolved the episodes of hypoglycemia. Although he requires life-long immunosuppressive therapy to "protect" the implanted stem cells from immune attack, he accepts this small price to pay for the incredible improvement in his life. This is a historic landmark achievement and has garnered widespread press, including in the *New York Times*. More patients are currently being enrolled in this study.

Dr. David Scadden at Harvard's Stem Cell Institute has cautioned us that there are additional hurdles on the horizon:

- The reprogrammed cells are not identical to the native cells and may have hidden dysfunctions.
- Cells grown in a cell culture for prolonged periods exhibit a "genetic instability" that we will need to ensure is not detrimental or dangerous and, if it is, to figure out ways to prevent it.
- Assessing the risk of stem cell therapy in humans will require years of clinical testing.

Clinical Trials

If you or a loved one has type 1 diabetes and are very keen to explore stem cell treatment, we suggest you approach a reputable academic center. If you are interested to enroll in a clinical trial, make sure that it is one that has been approved by the Institutional Review Board (IRB) to ensure that that safety and efficacy are being diligently monitored.

There are innumerable private clinics around the world making bold but unproven and even false claims about stem cell treatment and cashing in unscrupulously. Be prudent!

Key Points

- One of the challenges with stem cell transplantation in a patient with type 1 diabetes is that the immune system that attacked the beta cells in the first place will also attack the new beta cells. Researchers are currently working hard to address this problem.
- If you or a loved one has type 1 diabetes and are very keen to explore stem cell treatment, we suggest you approach a reputable academic center to enroll.

24

VACCINATIONS

Vaccinations simply save lives, from the newborn to old age.

—Sanjiv Chopra and Martin Abrahamson

According to the Centers for Disease Control and Prevention (CDC) patients with type 1 and type 2 diabetes may be at higher risk of acquiring infections that can be prevented through vaccination.

The CDC recommends that the following five vaccines be administered to patients with diabetes:

1. **Influenza**: Influenza can be a serious infection with significant morbidly and mortality. An *annual* flu shot is recommended.
2. **Pneumococcal**: Pneumococcal Disease can result in both pneumonia and meningitis. An initial vaccine and then a repeat dose five years later is recommended.
3. **Tdap**: This vaccine protects against tetanus, diphtheria, and pertussis (whooping cough). All three of these conditions can be serious and life-threatening. The tetanus and diphtheria vaccine should be given every ten years.
4. **Herpes Zoster (Shingles)**: This vaccine protects against shingles, which presents with a rash and pain. The pain can be debilitating, and last for months. A new vaccine requires two shots, the second dose being administered two to six months later.
5. **Hepatitis B Virus (HBV)**: Vaccination against HBV was first recommended by the CDC in 2011. It is recommended for people with diabetes between 19 and 60 years of age. Hepatitis B virus infection can be acute or chronic. Patients with chronic infection are at risk for developing cirrhosis, liver failure and cancer of the liver (see page 80). All patients with underlying chronic liver disease should receive both the Hepatitis A and Hepatitis B vaccines if a blood test indicates they do not have pre-existing immunity.

Vaccination guidelines are frequently updated. We recommend that you check with your primary care clinician to see that you are compliant with the latest recommendations.

25

A PRACTICAL CHECKLIST

The checklist is one of the most high-powered productivity tools ever discovered.

—Brian Tracy

To-do lists help us break life into small steps.

—Randy Pausch

When your next diabetes checkup isn't for another three, or possibly six months, you may find it hard to stay motivated in all aspects of your self-care. Below is a checklist that we hope will help.

Healthy Routines

Consider posting this on your fridge, bathroom mirror, or any place you will see each morning:

1. **Mindful eating**: Use a written diary or an app to help you record food to help you stay true to your goals. Remember that all the good things you are doing will pay handsome dividends in the long run!
2. **Exercise daily**: Walk briskly for 30 minutes or turn on the music and dance for 30 minutes or clean the house for 30 mins. The exercise that works best is the one that you enjoy doing. Remember that there is no "upper limit" to how much exercise you do each day!
3. **Test your blood sugars** every day or as often as recommended by your health care provider
4. **Medications**: Double check that you have taken **all** your medications – use weekly medication dispensers or an app to be sure that you have taken all your medications each day.
5. **Vaccinations**: Be current with your vaccination schedule (see page 215).

Preparing for the Consultation

To maximize the benefit of your visit with your clinician (in person or via telehealth):

- Upload or have available **glucose logs**, either in written form or available to be downloaded from a website, or from a glucose meter.
- Keep a **log of food and activity** for the preceding week. This will help your provider interpret the glucose data more effectively.
- Make a note if you have had any episodes of **hypoglycemia**, and if so, if you think there is anything that you did to cause this, e.g., did you take more insulin prior to the meal and then eat less? Did you exercise more or differently than usual?
- Be prepared to discuss **any problems** that might be concerning no matter how trivial you think they may be.

The Consultation

Your clinician should be asking if you have any major concerns at every visit. She or he should be reviewing your glucose monitoring data, medications, diet and exercise, inquiring about hypoglycemia, and ensuring that you are up to date with all of your required screening tests and vaccinations see below.

At every visit the following should be done:

1. **Height**, **weight**, and **blood pressure** should be checked.
2. The **thyroid gland** should be examined.
3. **Feet** should be examined.

On the following page, we provide a checklist that you can print out or copy. We recommend that you make a couple of printouts of this checklist. Keep one in your health folder and take one with you when you go to see your health care provider, so that everyone is on the same page.

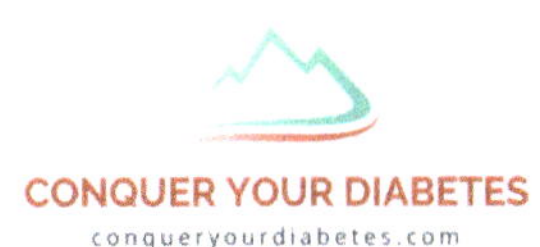

Diabetes Monitoring Checklist

At every visit:

1. Height, weight, and blood pressure.
2. Thyroid gland examination.
3. Feet examination.

EVERY 3–6 MONTHS

(6- monthly if well-controlled)

☐ **Hemoglobin A1c** 1) 2) ________________

Dates

3)________________

YEARLY

☐ **Cholesterol profile** ________________ *Date*

☐ **Kidney function tests** ________________ *Date*

☐ **Urine microalbumin** ________________ *Date*

☐ **Liver function tests** ________________ *Date*

☐ **Thyroid function tests (TSH)** ________________ *Date*

☐ **Eye examination by an ophthalmologist** *At time of diagnosis and annually thereafter (type 2 diabetes); annually after 5 years of type 1 diabetes.* ________________ *Date*

Allow the teachings to enter you as you might listen to music or as in the way the earth allows rain to permeate it.

—Thich Nhat Hanh

Useful Resources

We recommend the following resources for further information on diabetes and its management:

- American Diabetes Association – https://www.diabetes.org/.
- Association of Diabetes Care and Education Specialists – https://www.diabeteseducator.org/.
- International Diabetes Federation – https://idf.org/.
- Endocrine Society – https://www.endocrine.org/.
- American Association Study for the study of Liver Diseases (AASLD) – https://www.aasld.org/.
- UpToDate - https://www.uptodate.com.
- American Heart Association – https://www.heart.org/.
- Centers for Disease Control and Prevention – https://www.cdc.gov/diabetes/basics/diabetes.html.

Index

D

www.ingramcontent.com/pod-product-compliance
Ingram Content Group UK Ltd.
Pitfield, Milton Keynes, MK11 3LW, UK
UKHW062303290726
14090UKWH00017B/852

9 798985 423716